Family Kaleidoscope

Family Kaleidoscope

Salvador Minuchin

Harvard University Press

Cambridge, Massachusetts, and London, England

To my mother and to my aunts Sofia and Esther,
who also mothered me

Library of Congress Cataloging in Publication Data
Minuchin, Salvador.
  Family kaleidoscope.
  Bibliography: p.
  1. Family psychotherapy—Miscellanea. 2. Family—
United States—Anecdotes, facetiae, satire, etc.
3. Minuchin, Salvador. 4. Psychotherapists—United
States—Biography. I. Title.
RC488.5.M557 1984   616.89′156   84-9140
ISBN 0-674-29230-8 (alk. paper) (cloth)
ISBN 0-674-29231-6 (paper)

Acknowledgments

This book owes a great deal to many people, in many countries, since several of the chapters were written as part of my peripatetic teaching over the past few years. Let me start off by thanking Fred Gottlieb, who suggested the title—titles have always been a problem for me. Donald Bloch and Edna Shapiro read the manuscript and gave me many valuable suggestions.

"Trio" is a family that was part of a research project on families of divorce done at the Philadelphia Child Guidance Clinic, and I want to thank Marla Isaacs there. Nan Lombaers invited me to see the commune in Holland during the late sixties; I discussed "The Key" with her when I began to write it and am grateful for her input. My London "Day in Court" owes much to Alan Cooklin, director of the Marlborough Day Hospital, and to the staff of that hospital. Gill Gorell-Barnes gave me a good deal of the literature portraying child abuse in England, and we discussed the case of Maria Colwell and the possibility (which we never developed) of making a follow-up study of Maria's siblings. Irene Levin in Norway translated the transcript of the Andersson sessions and provided both follow-up and many helpful comments on the case. I want to thank Eleanor Bron for encouraging me to transform my clinical experience into the play form.

Marge Arnold's loyalty and hard work during the writing of this book made the whole project possible. Fran Hitchcock has continued to help me recast my thinking into readable English. I would also like to thank Joyce Backman for her editing, and of course my wife Pat, with whom I check all my half-formed ideas to gain the courage to go ahead with them.

Contents

Introduction

It is 8 a.m. The TV is tuned to the local public broadcasting station, and the face of a two-week-old baby appears on the screen. A large card with brightly colored concentric circles is held in front of the child. As it moves slowly toward her, her arms move forward and her head arches back. The commentator, a casually dressed psychologist from the university, tells the audience that we have underestimated the human infant's repertory of responses. He makes a loud noise to show the infant's startle response, which is clearly different from her attempt to defend herself from the advancing circles.

The commentator goes on to explain that in the last decade information about infants' capacities has mushroomed. Many psychologists have presented infants with simple stimuli and have recorded their complex sets of responses. Slowly our understanding of an extraordinary organism—the average human being at birth—has increased and evolved, and now movies and related technologies are transforming clinicians' dry language into a heart-melting dialog between the exploring infant on the screen and an entranced audience.

But the average human being at birth does not live in the organized simplicity of a psychology laboratory. The baby is born into a family, and any mental-health technician will agree as to the importance of that fact. There exploration seems to stop.

We know so much about the individual—shouldn't we know more about the family? Well, of course. On the other hand, surely we are all experts. We grew up as part of a family organism, and many of us repeat and improve on familiar experience. We have children of our own. Immediately we are in trouble. Our parenting seems to be an exercise of moving by approximation from mistake to mistake. We fumble, hope, improve, compromise, and despair in different ratios according to our different styles. No one else seems to have such difficulty: other parents know how to do it right. *Their* lives are ordered; *their* children's problems are intelligently handled. So what's wrong with us?

I've been a family therapist for over thirty years and can't begin to guess how many families I've met. Never have I met a parent who isn't sure that other parents handle things more smoothly. Everyone knows other families' problems are well handled and logically resolved. My own parents knew it, and so do my children. The well-functioning "typical American family" continues to be a staple of movies, magazines, and television. At some level everyone knows it's a myth, but the myth is destructive because, as our own experience inevitably falls short, our best efforts seem to be failures.

Why is our image of the ideal family so far from the common reality? We are a culture that has enthroned the individual. We have an extraordinarily rich literature of individual psychology, but our insight has focused on the being inside of the self. This is an extraordinary feat of the imagination because "decontexted" individuals do not exist. Life consists of growing, mixing, cooperating, sharing, and competing with others. Surely most of us have had our most significant experiences within some form of the complex social unit we call a family. Why is this social organism invisible to our experts? Why isn't it represented in legislatures? Why doesn't it have legal counsel in the courts?

The answers are embedded in history, politics, and economics. They are worth exploring, for as we study why the family is invisible, we begin to understand why psychology and ethnology understand territoriality and aggression better than sharing and cooperation, though there are innumerable examples of both. Exploring the enthroning of the individual illuminates why economics so often deals with the maximum utilization of resources instead of their interrelation. And why even our "family" courts deal with confrontation rather than mutuality.

We have the capacity for more accurate perceptions of human

reality: after all, when we are shown a mouth and eyes in a gestalt perception test, we recognize a face. The same capacity might enable us to look at an individual and recognize a family. But the paradigms of our culture betray us with a trompe l'oeil: the whole is distorted through emphasis on the detail.

This book is an attempt to help you see differently. Not necessarily better, but differently. Most of us are like Molière's "bourgeois gentilhomme," who had been speaking prose all his life and never knew it. We live our lives like chips in a kaleidoscope, always part of patterns that are larger than ourselves and somehow more than the sum of their parts. Our individual epistemology usually blinds us to this kaleidoscopic self, and that is unfortunate because, when we look at human beings from this perspective, whole new possibilities open up for exploring behavior and alleviating pain.

In one way and another, I have been working to define the message of this book throughout my whole professional career. But I think it relevant to point out that this particular statement springs from a specific period in my life. Two years ago my wife and I began a new chapter: we took early retirement. Both of us, though still enjoying the challenge of teaching others, had the frustrating feeling that we ourselves were learning less. After much discussion we decided to take a year off to live in London. Settled there, we followed a lifelong interest in normal families and pursued the study of the processes of divorce and remarriage. Pat began to play the oboe. I toyed with writing plays. It was a period to experiment with being inexpert and to follow whatever intellectual pathway chance threw our way.

For a while it felt strange not to have to respond to the constraints and demands of university and clinic. Separated from the structuring of a daily schedule, I suffered many periods of uncertainty that I had avoided by feeling effective as a teacher and practitioner of family therapy. Then rather suddenly I realized I was seeing things differently. No longer having to concentrate on how to help the Smith family change, I was able to ask myself how Smith families function and how they work within the social context. No longer forced to respond to the immediacies of executive or administrative tasks, I began to ask deeper, more generic, questions. Not how to do therapy, but how do families work? Not what are the best training curricula, but have family therapists achieved a paradigmatic change in the organization of institutions that deal with people? Long a member of the councils of family therapy, I began to feel like an Elder in those councils. With this new freedom came new responsibilities—the need to look at the tribe as a whole.

Without conscious awareness, I began to reexamine the problems that led me to family therapy thirty years ago—the workings of families with delinquent children. In that other country (and in so many ways, another era), I returned to family court to resume the exploration of families of the slums. But now, after so many years of accepting the way institutions label families and taking families on the institutions' terms, I wanted to explore what institutions do to families.

So this book is, in a sense, an interim report, growing out of a pause in the life of an intervener. Maybe what it really is is a travelog: I've been traveling through family country; I'd like to show you some sights. Or perhaps there is only one area, which displays its varying textures as we circle around it. It seems to me that all I want to do is show how the reality of human nature goes beyond the individual as a complete system. When I talk about divorce, remarriage, family therapy, the judiciary, the medical system, and violence in families, I am always telling the same story.

The itinerary I have set is a trifle arbitrary, very personal. The book is divided into sections containing a potpourri of cases, dialogs, discussions, fables, and plays. I have mixed fact and fiction with no real attempt to sort them out in the usual scholarly fashion. Each claims to portray reality—just as in life.

Part One

Patterns in
Transition

Kaleidoscope

Fragments

Looking into the interior of a family, one can suddenly be caught by scenarios. These may be whimsical, challenging, absurd, or dramatic, but they are all disturbing because they carry the tantalizing feeling that they are complete. It is as if one glanced into a store window, and flashed the universe.

But the truth is that the family therapist is always in the presence of shifting images. Often he focuses on one well-defined piece—the family's presentation of their identified patient. But there are hundreds of other pieces with clear or uneven edges that have to be fitted together in order to see the pattern, and perhaps change the position of the pieces.

What follows are two puzzles, pieced together to show you how the game is played.

The Magdalene

I met the Flauberts in Europe. They had requested therapy and accepted the offer of an initial session with me and the psychiatrist who would then continue treating them.

As I first saw them in the office of the family therapist, the father, an official of a foreign embassy, seemed an escapee from the pages of John le Carré: dark glasses, a beret that he kept on, gray flannel trousers and a blue blazer, a high-necked blue shirt, and a paperback book on structuralism in his hand. The mother, also in her forties, was a study in dignified femininity with an aura of Chanel No. 5 and English knitwear. Their daughter Cecily was clearly claiming that she belonged to another family, in a world of the uninhibited whose uniforms are colorful, wrinkled, and frayed.

Sophisticated makeup hid her fourteen-year-old innocence—though she would probably scorn the word; for the last six months she had been taking a different man to bed almost every night. She always managed to leave clues for her parents to find. They had suspected and at first denied the facts. Then, unable to lie any longer to themselves or each other, they had confronted her. Her answer was that genuine challenge of the young: "So what?" The lines had been drawn—on one side the parents, filled with impotent rage and hidden guilt, on the other the girl, with all the power of the helpless. She had come at her mother's insistence, resolved not to say anything: her parents might drag her to the psychiatrist, but they could not make her drink.

At the beginning of the session, as usual, there were a lot of irrelevant movements, as if bodies had to find the right spot on the chairs or the most protected corner. Then there was an exchange of looks, from father to mother, mother to daughter and therapist, the girl to her hands. All were fast enough to avoid detection—nobody wanted to be the family informer.

I began some irrelevant comments on the weather, traffic conditions, the TV camera in the corner. This is the social gambit: white pawn/king nine. The father responded in kind, black pawn/king three. Casually I asked, "Who would like to tell me why you're here today?" A fast exchange of messages between the parents resulted in the mother's taking the voice for the family. I acknowledged the expected move; it usually is the mother. The question of who will begin is part of an informal guessing game I enjoy: Will the man ask the woman to talk, or will she start straight away?

MOTHER: Well, we came because Cecily is acting strangely. No, not strangely, but certainly it's not characteristic. She's always been a very good student. She's very bright, and she was very hard-working, but this semester she's failing almost all her subjects.

CECILY: I am not!

MOTHER: You told me you're failing math and history. Isn't that true?

CECILY: Forget it!
MOTHER: If I'm misquoting you, just tell me.

Silence fell—back to square one. The father rearranged his dark glasses. I had a strange impulse to pull them away to see if there was a man there. I acknowledged the feeling, suppressed the impulse, and looked expectantly at the mother.

MOTHER: You know we love you, Cecily, and we came here to help you. But if you don't talk, we're helpless.
CECILY: I said forget it!
MINUCHIN: Would you mind, Cecily, if your mother or father tells me why you are all here? You can correct them if they're not accurate.
CECILY: I don't mind.
M: Would you prefer your father or your mother?
CECILY: I don't care.

I was treading softly, trying to keep the door open. The mother had said over the phone that they were concerned about Cecily's promiscuity and that they suspected she had been "selling her body." Her opening, talking about school, was one of the meandering ways by which frightened parents approach problems.

M: Mr. Flaubert, would you like to tell me how you see the problem?
FATHER (*puts his book on a nearby table, takes his glasses and beret off with the same movement, and puts them down—a man after all, and a worried one*): Let's cut it out, Lydia. We all know why we're here. Cecily hasn't slept in her bed for weeks. She leaves home before I get back from the embassy, and returns at three or four in the morning. She sleeps all day, and she's been cutting school for the last month. (*He doesn't look at either Cecily or me while he talks. His wife is the target, and he spits his words out with contained anger. He shifts in the chair, pulls up his pants before crossing his legs, then looks directly at me.*) I learned all this three days ago—from the school principal. She called me at the embassy.
MOTHER: I didn't want to tell you because I was afraid of what you'd do to her.

FATHER: What could I do? Shoot her?

MOTHER: I was afraid.

M: Excuse me. How long has this been going on?

MOTHER: For quite a while, but it's been increasing this last month.

M: And you learned all of this only three days ago, Mr. Flaubert? I don't understand that.

FATHER: Lydia has been protecting her. I leave home at six in the morning and I come back late. Cecily's been angry at me for the last month and she's been avoiding me. I thought her need for distance was a necessary part of growing up, and I accepted it. (*In an incongruous gesture, he puts his dark glasses on again. I wonder if he's signaling his disappearance.*)

M: Is your father a very violent man, Cecily? Or is your mother protecting you because she doesn't think you're grown up?

CECILY: She thinks I'm ten years old! She talks about me as if I'm six. We can't get together at all; we just talk *at* each other. And my father doesn't talk at all. He just hides behind his important books and his dark glasses.

It would be difficult for any adolescent to resist an invitation to explore parental failures. Cecily's answer reveals a bright and bitter girl, skillful in using words. I guess she is caught in some struggle between her parents, and bent on self-destruction.

At certain points in a session I let family members talk, encouraging their interaction, and I float. That way I can get some perspective on the whole family organism. For the Flauberts, I sense the father's fear of being discovered, the mother's dignified aloofness, and Cecily's despair, commingling in a dance of tenuous contact. In the computer of my brain, with its billions of connections, images come and go—checked, connected, replaced, retrieved. I think, without thinking, about the mother's possible lovers, the father's machismo or homosexuality, Cecily's feelings of betrayal: chips of eidetic information form the uneasy background against which I explore further.

M: I'm quite impressed, Mr. Flaubert, that important events can occur in your house without your knowledge. I see, by the way, you're reading Foucault. He's remarkable. I think he takes the truth and turns it on its head. Well . . . how is it possible, Mr. Flaubert, that you didn't know?

FATHER: My wife left us three days ago.

I don't make a move. My eyes unfocus in my best imitation of the invisible man. This is a time to wait.

MOTHER: It's true. But I waited around long enough—a doormat for you to wipe your intellectual feet on! I was a nothing, thinking I had to sacrifice myself for Cecily's sake, all my life, just waiting! I'm forty-five. I need to be myself. Now!

All the forces contained in twenty years of marriage collide here at accelerating speeds. Their story is not so special, as they tell it. They were always mismatched: Maurice the only son of an academic couple, shy and intellectual, pursuing a career; Lydia a child of the bourgeoisie, marrying above her station and organizing her life to advance her husband's career. She wanted many children; they had only one. Cecily became her mother's project, then her friend, and finally her confidante. Everything was routine until a couple of years ago, when Lydia, with her child growing up, decided to study for a degree. Maurice supported her decision, and Cecily felt it was fun to have a mother at the university.

FATHER: I really want you to come back. Of course you have the right to decide—but we need you.

MOTHER: I don't think you need me, Maurice. I don't think you even noticed when I left . . . well, maybe that's unfair. But I really think you'll manage.

CECILY: What about me? I suppose I'm supposed to manage too?

MOTHER: I want you to come live with me. I told you that.

FATHER: No! I don't want that. Cecily already has a home. It's your home too, but apparently you've decided to leave it. We'll manage. (*He looks at Cecily.*) I'll have to get to know you better.

Triangulation is a dirty game, but family members play it frequently. Children have to find their own way, and Cecily, at fourteen, is reasonably well equipped to make some decisions. But there is a quirk in this situation.

M: You're in a very difficult spot, Cecily, but I think your solution is self-destructive. To go whoring because your parents split up is not very smart.

CECILY: I'm not a whore! I just don't want to be home. I have a lot of friends, and we go out together—

FATHER: And you stay out till four in the morning.

MOTHER: You could stay with me.

CECILY: And Bella?

M: Who is Bella?

FATHER: Her lover. Lydia not only left me . . . she's decided she's a lesbian.

We had been together almost an hour, and this was a scenario I had not foreseen. I had speculated that the father might be impotent, that he might be a homosexual, that the mother might have a lover, but a woman lover had not occurred to me. It struck me how bound I was to surfaces. Lydia was a very attractive woman, sending distinctly feminine vibes. Out of my own confusion, I could understand Cecily's frenzied destructiveness.

M: Do you know Bella, Cecily?

CECILY: She was Mother's best friend, and my friend too. She's divorced, and she's been a lesbian for years.

M: So you really feel betrayed.

CECILY: Yes, I do. My mother shouldn't have done that.

M: What do you mean by "that"? (*I indicate that she should talk with her mother about it.*)

CECILY: You shouldn't have left us.

MOTHER (*gently*): I don't think you can understand.

CECILY: I understand it's rotten!

MOTHER: But you know I was very unhappy. You know Daddy and I don't get along. It's different with Bella. It might seem strange to you, but we really love each other.

CECILY: You're just talking about screwing!

FATHER: Cecily! Don't talk like that to your mother!

And here they were, caught in conventions—and deviation, confusion, and pain.

MOTHER: Do you know what screwing really is, Cecily?
CECILY: Yes I do. It's not so special. Lots of times it's just exercise.

Poor Cecily. At fourteen . . .
The session, run by the clock, not by family dynamics or level of pain, was over. My colleague made arrangements for the next session. In leaving this family I said something "deep," asking Cecily if she knew her promiscuity was to reassure herself that she was a woman. Child-adult that she was, she simply said yes. I asked her why she was doing it. "For punishment," she laughed shortly. I did not ask for whom.

The Healer

Another time I found myself supervising a young psychologist. I sat behind a one-way mirror, and we agreed that I would telephone the therapist whenever I had a suggestion about his conduct of the interview.

The mother was the first to enter the interview room, then the father, and their children Jane and Eddie. Through the one-way mirror I watched Eddie, aged eleven. His whole demeanor demanded attention: his shuffling walk, the droop of his head as he studied the wall-to-wall carpet that covered the interview room. In the doorway he managed to step on his untied shoelaces and catapult into the room. After he regained his balance his arms resumed their gangling droop. He conveyed a strange mixture of depression and incompetence that might elicit pity or laughter, depending on your degree of detachment.

Jane, two years older and taller, with big blue eyes that studied the room with frank interest, seemed efficient and effective, a typical bright teenager. Clearly she felt sure of herself.

Eddie opened the session with a whimper. I strained to hear but had to turn up the audio. His complaint had to do with failing in his chores at home, for which his father had fined him two dollars. The father, a rather thin, wiry man, explained to Eddie that he thought he'd done well in many of the chores, but that once he'd failed in one he had had no choice but to cut Eddie's allowance. He was careful to say that he loved Eddie and repeated that the boy had done well in the other chores. His voice took on a strange quiver as he attempted the complex task of maintaining his decision without hurting Eddie's self-esteem.

The therapist had told me that this was his third session with the family. They had come to therapy because of Eddie's depression, his crying spells, his isolation in school. The therapist was impressed by the parents' overinvolvement with the children and their lack of competence in parenting. Both father and mother seemed to be in a constant state of hyperalertness, ready to cushion the floor before the children fell down. Jane never did, but Eddie could keep them busy full time.

The young psychologist thought it was necessary to create some distance between parents and children, and to give the parents a chance to observe before they took protective action. Trained in behavioral techniques, he had convinced the parents of the significance of Parent Effectiveness Techniques, taught them how to make charts, and showed them the system of accounting that records rewards and punishments.

The results were marvelous: the family had arrived at this session transformed. The parents, armed with a new way of looking, and enchanted with all the dotted *i*'s and crossed *t*'s, had become clearer in their demands and, though somewhat tyrannical, were at least predictable. Jane was glowing with all her gold stars, and Eddie's whimpering had at least become more concrete: he had tried but failed, and received demerits. But now in a very low voice, with tears in his eyes, he was saying the program was unfair, that they should have been allowed some trial runs in the beginning before they were evaluated.

THERAPIST: Eddie, that's very good! Can you convince your parents?
EDDIE (*studying the floor, sniffing audibly*): No.
THERAPIST: Are they very rigid, Eddie? Who is stricter?
EDDIE: My dad.
FATHER: Why do you think so, Eddie? You know I'm fair, and I love you. You washed the dishes very well last night, and you made your bed this morning. I gave you two points each time. You lost points because you didn't put out the trash, but—

Eddie reinforced his father's attention with more silent tears. The mother, her body stretched toward her son, began talking to him. The therapist made a gesture indicating that this was between Eddie and his father; she stopped in mid-sentence. Marveling at the efficiency of Eddie's silence, I rang the therapist and suggested that he try to engage Eddie and Jane in a sibling coalition to confront their parents. He said okay, sat silent, thinking a moment, and then as if it had just come to him:

THERAPIST: Eddie, maybe you can convince Jane. I think you have a very good point. If you can convince her, maybe between the two of you, you can change your parents' view.

EDDIE (*his voice somewhat louder*): Do you think they should give us another chance?

JANE: I'm doing all right, but if you want . . . I think that would be fair. They could give us some chances before a new task.

EDDIE: But they don't think it's necessary.

JANE: If we talk with Dad I think he'll agree.

THERAPIST: Who's harder to convince, Eddie?

EDDIE (*whimpering again*): My dad.

THERAPIST: Who do you think, Jane?

JANE: My mom.

THERAPIST (*to children*): Stand up (*he stands in front of them*). Eddie, what grade are you in?

EDDIE: Seventh.

THERAPIST: Jane?

JANE: Freshman.

THERAPIST: Eddie, I'm really surprised. You're almost as tall as your sister, and you're very bright. But you still keep, inside yourself, a little, crying voice that is six years old. How did you manage that? In your family, who's helped you keep that?

Bull's eye! I like this dance. The therapist, abandoning his behavioral approach, is moving with the family now, accommodating to their movements, anticipating them, and starting to lead the family.

JANE: I think it was Mom.

THERAPIST: How? Could you tell me, Jane?

JANE: I think she worries a lot for him.

THERAPIST (*to parents*): You have a future psychologist at home. Congratulations! (*Jane and mother laugh.*)

This is a noteworthy move. Anticipating a challenge to the mother, the therapist congratulates her for having a smart daughter, confirming her before the challenge.

THERAPIST: Do you agree with my future colleague?
MOTHER: Yes. I do overprotect him.
THERAPIST: How?
FATHER: We all do it. We're a family of saviors.

Father's comment is a protective maneuver. I enjoy the aesthetic precision of this family's dance.

The mother describes Eddie's childhood. His fear of strangers started when he was four months old, much sooner than Dr. Spock's norms. Even his own grandparents frightened him; he would cling to his mother, and she held him tightly, feeling his little body relax. It was a wonderful feeling for her to experience this ability to shield him against the frightening world. I think of the many times I have seen this mythmaking: parents forming the future behavior of a child, projecting their dreams, fears, and expectations onto him. Why and how was this fear created? What is its symbolic meaning? What patterns of family life are contained in the mother's projection?

THERAPIST: Eddie, do you think you could help your mother relax now? The way she helped you relax when you were an infant?
EDDIE (*looking at mother*): What do I have to do to convince you that I can do things?

This is an interesting twist. Maintaining the theme of helpfulness that seems so important in this family of rescuers, the therapist has changed the direction of the function, and Eddie has assumed a competent role. Eddie looks more like an average eleven-year-old now.

FATHER: I think I'm the cause of Eddie's fears. I really don't know whether it has anything to do with Eddie's depression, or whatever you call it. But when Eddie was born—almost the same time—they discovered that I had cancer of the colon, and I had my first operation.

Suddenly father and mother were describing their lives in those years: intermittent hospitalizations, sometimes lasting months, four abdominal operations, chemotherapy, periods of remission and optimism, days of despair. The mother talked about her effort to maintain sanity, hiding her feelings, not crying—the nervous breakdown that hospitalized *her* for three months. While the parents described ten years of living with death, Eddie returned to his examination of the carpet. Jane's blue eyes stared unfocusing into the one-way mirror.

I called the therapist to join me behind the looking glass. Eddie's symptoms could be seen from the perspective of their function in a family that was struggling with death (or was it life?). The mother's protection when he was an infant had helped her feel competent when she helplessly thought her husband was dying. Later, concentrating on Eddie had given both parents a detour from their depressing reality.

The question, of course, was: Were Eddie's payments necessary to his family's balance? We didn't think so. I suggested that the therapist meet with the parents alone, request permission to talk to the father's oncologist, find out as much as he could about the father's prognosis, and, if he thought it useful, invite the doctor to a session. After a couple of sessions, the therapist might begin to alternate between the couple and the family as a whole, focusing on how to live in the present instead of mourning the future. Perhaps Eddie could continue to be a family healer without also having to be its sacrificial lamb.

READER: You know, I find these vignettes rather interesting. But for me, the drama is still centered on the transformation of meaning going on in Cecily and Eddie.

AUTHOR: Now you see how difficult it is to move away from the perspective of the individual. I am writing this book to make you see differently.

READER: Then you'll have to do better. Compared with the deep mysteries of the Magdalene's psyche, the transactions between her and her parents are totally flat. They're manipulating each other, but so what? All that does is reinforce my concern for the survival of the individual caught so helplessly in the family web.

AUTHOR: But the individual is also the web. How can I communicate something that is so self-evident?

READER: Self-evident? The family that I see—

AUTHOR: But you see only what fits your models. And since your cognitive models of reality spring from an egocentric point of view—"I looking at the world"—you see the family only as an envelope.

READER: And you're going to convince me that your point of view is better?

AUTHOR: Not necessarily. But I will attempt to challenge your certainty.

READER: How? I know what I see.

AUTHOR: By showing you what you have made invisible.

READER: That sounds obscure enough to be tantalizing.

AUTHOR: Far from it. You are, like "the Magdalene" and "the Healer," one well-defined piece in a pattern that you don't see.

READER: If I'm so blind, how can *you* be so all-seeing?

AUTHOR: I don't call you blind for not seeing what is not there to see.

READER: Mysticism, now?

AUTHOR: No, difficulty. You see, it really is impossible for an individual to conceive that the whole of his being is only a part of larger organisms.

READER: That sounds like . . . religion? Physics? The unity of the Cosmos?

AUTHOR: Those are all cop-outs. It's easy to talk of oneself as part of something so large, distant, and noble. It's much more difficult to recognize yourself as part of a family pattern.

READER: All right, go ahead. How will you make the invisible appear?

AUTHOR: By letting you look into families in transition.

READER: Transition between what and what?

AUTHOR: Families have stages of life when they function without major upheaval. During these stages family members interact within a routine that is predictable—so predictable that it renders the family as an organism invisible. To see the family, you have to look at it as it is in motion—changing from one form to another.

READER: I think I follow you. At certain periods, the idiosyncratic movements of each family member can be seen as part of a larger design. Something like a ballet? A jam session?

AUTHOR: Or a Greek tragedy, or Pirandello's *Six Characters,* or the wholeness of ecological niches . . .

READER: That's a major task. Do you have a plan of attack?

AUTHOR: We'll look at three organisms. The first is moving from a nuclear family into a divorced family. The second is a divorced family moving into a blended shape. The third is a commune experiencing the dissolution of its group. In each case the organism will show itself as its members search for new blue-prints that will allow it to function with economy while changing.

Trio

Patterns of Divorce

As the divorce rate has increased in the United States, we have seen a concomitant rise in the number of cooperative separations. Spouses contemplating a divorce explore its consequences to their parental functions. Many decide that while they want to stop affiliating as spouses, they want to continue cooperating as parents. I know of one instance in which the divorced spouses remained in the same house (a rather large one), dividing their space, and continued to parent their children in an expanded family that ultimately included their new partners and their children—a rather cumbersome arrangement that nonetheless exemplifies the freedom to innovate away from our old nuclear family model.

The period after the separation is always stressful for family members. They must negotiate new patterns of functioning while the blueprints that governed the old family still control their habitual responses. Family therapists who see families in the period of transition may misdiagnose the search for new patterns and the ensuing pain. We may label as deviant what is actually the creative attempt of a family organism to develop a new shape—the shedding and becoming that precede a butterfly.

We need to explore separation and divorce so as to develop ways of helping family members move from one pattern to another. As a step in such exploration, I interviewed the Jansons. At the first interview, the spouses had been separated for over a year and were in the process of divorcing. The two daughters, Natalie, thirteen, and Vicky, ten, had remained with their mother, but visited their father most weekends. The second interview occurred eighteen months later, two years after the father's departure. The interviews were framed as explorations of normal family functioning, and the Jansons were paid a small fee for their participation.

MINUCHIN: So, you understand the purpose of the meeting. I want to explore the ways in which your family has changed since Mr. Janson left the house. Is it okay if I start with the children? (*Mother nods.*) Your name is Vicky, is that right? How has life changed now that you're three people instead of four?

VICKY: Well, I guess—it seems that my sister and I get into fights more than we used to. We can't get as many things because my father's not living with us. So we can't buy as much, and stuff like that.

MOTHER: How has life changed for you in particular?

VICKY: Well, I've changed schools. And we might have to move.

M: Why is that?

VICKY: Because my dad doesn't live with us. The house is big, and . . .

M: And that will be a problem for you?

VICKY: Yes. All my friends live here.

M: How about your mom? Will it be a problem for her?

VICKY: Yes. Her friends live here too.

M: Can you think of any other change?

VICKY: Well, I guess not.

MOTHER: How about feeling insecure about what's going to happen to us?

VICKY: Well . . .

MOTHER: About the future, what's going to happen.

It seems likely that the mother is expressing her own concerns, inducing a parallel mood in the child. Since all family members, experiencing the stress of transition, try to draw closer together, the family becomes a resonating box where one member's insecurity reverberates through the other family members.

VICKY: Since my dad left I always get the feeling that my mom might leave too.

M: That's an interesting thought. It seems rather strange to me, though. Why would your mom leave?

VICKY: I figure my dad left, so my mom can leave too.

M: Your dad left because he and your mom had some issues to resolve. Did he divorce you too?

VICKY: Really he didn't. He just left my mom. He really didn't leave us. Just her.

M: He left your mom and your mom left him.

VICKY: Yes. But it seems like he left us.

While the Jansons have given Vicky the explanations parents usually give to their children—we are divorcing, but we'll still be your parents—Vicky's experiential reality is that her father divorced her as well. This type of experience varies, of course, in different families, but for younger children the difficult and confusing experience often leads to fantasies of abandonment. For the Janson children, the expression of these fantasies is not the product of amorphous anxiety. It is a chip in the poker game all children play with their parents, sometimes with painful skill. It's a way of manipulating Mother, ever so slightly tightening the noose.

M: And now you think that maybe Mom could leave you too?

VICKY: Yes.

M: Why would that be? Natalie, do you think so too? (*Natalie nods.*) Okay, talk together. What do you do to your mom, that you think she'll leave you?

VICKY: Well, she gets upset if we fight with each other. And we're always fighting.

Simple events that before would only have brought fear of increased discipline become part of abandonment fantasies.

M: Talk to Natalie about that. Your mother and I will listen.

NATALIE: Oh well, we always fight. She hates that. And we get mad at her. We cry quite often. We aggravate her.

VICKY: Well, I was thinking—because of Dad, I was scared that she might go away. Like Dad.

NATALIE: She could find someone else to replace us. She wouldn't need us any more. She'd have someone else.

M: Does she have a boyfriend?

NATALIE: Yes—Mike.

M: And you think the boyfriend could replace you?

NATALIE and VICKY: Yes.

M: But I would assume that her relationship with Mike would be different from her relationship with you. Or does she mother him?

VICKY (*laughing*): No.

M: Then how could he replace you? That's kind of interesting.

VICKY: Well, not replace us, but—like, if he spends more time with her than we do, she might forget about us. Well, not forget about us, but just spend more time with him. Spend more and more time with him and not spend a lot of time with us.

In this transitional stage as the family members are developing patterns that will underpin their shape as a trio, the mother's new boyfriend is experienced by the children as a threat. Their response to this family change has been different because they are at different developmental stages. Natalie, a teenager, is exploring the possibilities of distancing by increasing her proximity to her adolescent friends. Vicky, at ten, needs closer proximity to her mother. To her, Mike is an intruder. I keep my questions in a light vein, in order to normalize their fear of abandonment and their aggressive fantasies.

M: I hope you've tried to distract your mom by fighting, so she doesn't forget you.

NATALIE: I don't think so.

M: Well, what kind of techniques do you use so your mom won't forget you?

NATALIE: We talk to her.

VICKY: Yes, we talk to her.

M: Do you tell her that you're afraid she'll put all her attention on Mike? What does she say? Does she reassure you?

NATALIE and VICKY: Yes.

M: How?

NATALIE: She says no matter how much Mike means to her, we mean a lot to her too.

M: But you still see Mike as keeping Mom's interest more than you would like?

VICKY: Yeah.

M: But that could be helpful, you know. Who needs Mom on your back all the time?

NATALIE (*laughing*): That's true.

M: Maybe it's different for you, Natalie. Maybe you don't need Mom now as much as Vicky does. What do you think?

VICKY: I don't think she does. She has all her friends—well, she has a best friend, Elizabeth. She's always over at her house.

M: So that means Natalie is abandoning Mom?

VICKY: Well, not abandoning her. But Elizabeth's always over. They're always together.

NATALIE: I'm over at Elizabeth's house or she's at our house.

M: And what about you?

VICKY: I have a friend, but not as close as Natalie and Elizabeth.

M: Let me ask you something, Natalie. Did Vicky begin to dress more like a grown-up in the last year?

I was impressed by the girls' clothing when they entered the office. Natalie was in the adolescent uniform: frayed jeans. But ten-year-old Vicky wore stockings and high heels. Her nails were polished, and her face was carefully made up. She seemed to be masquerading as an adult.

NATALIE: More like a grown-up?

M: You know, I look at you and I say you're a teenager. I look at Vicky and I think she's thirty-four.

NATALIE (*laughing*): Well yes, I think she dresses more grown-up.

M: I'm just curious about when she started to dress like that.

NATALIE: I don't remember. Maybe a couple of months ago.

M: When did you begin to dress so ladylike, Vicky?

VICKY: Oh, a couple of months ago.

M: When did you begin to wear stockings?

VICKY: I always wear them with a dress or a skirt. Except when I was little.

M (*to mother*): Did Vicky begin to dress more grown-up recently? Had you noticed that?

MOTHER: I didn't notice her wanting to be more grown-up. But I would say that in the past six months she's become a lot more conscious about her appearance in general.

M: How long have you been going with Mike?

MOTHER: Since last year. About eight months.

M: Because I was just wondering, Vicky, if you began to dress like a thirty-year-old woman when you thought that Mom might go live with Mike. Did you think you'd need to be grown-up then?

VICKY: I don't think so.

This focus on Vicky might be misconstrued as an exploration of some underlying problem. I decide to change focus and move toward the mother.

M: I was just curious. What are the changes that have occurred in your life—your name is Margaret?

MOTHER: Peg. I've had to become more independent financially. I worked for quite a while, but now I really have to work.

M: You work full time?

MOTHER: Yes. So I've become more aware of finances, and how much I need to work. I've become more independent in general. I had to find new friends, new activities—I guess in general to adjust to being a single parent.

M: It's a big adjustment.

MOTHER: Yes, it is. But I've become more adventurous. I guess I feel I don't have anybody to hold me back. There's nobody I have to confer with if I want to go some place or do something.

In the marriage, personal characteristics have to be modified or shed to conform to the complementarity of a couple. Returning to singlehood may have the effect of rediscovering the individual tempo. At the same time, parenting functions may become more difficult when the whole burden must be carried by a single parent. Yet they are also simpler because parenting has been disengaged from the negotiation of spouses who have different perspectives.

M: What about the children?

MOTHER: I'll confer with them. But I don't ask them if it's okay to do something. If it causes a big problem, then we'll discuss it and I might change my plans. But I don't think I ever have.

M: When you said confer with them, you looked at Natalie but not at Vicky. Do you see Natalie as the person with whom you check? More than Vicky?

MOTHER: Probably, yes. There's been a problem with Vicky. Or she sees it as a problem. I leave her out of discussions. I don't tell her things that . . . I know I'm wrong.

M: So it seems, Vicky, that Natalie has become a little like a friend of your mom's. That leaves you out.

VICKY: Not really a friend. Well, she tells Natalie more things than she tells me sometimes.

New families feel the ghosts of old structures like amputees experiencing their ghost limbs. For Peg, her husband's absence has left vacant a position for dialog. Natalie is moving into that position. I think the subsystem of separated spouse and one child is a typical transitional structure. It has stresses for all family members, but it also stretches capability. Natalie exercises new executive functioning, learning how to share and communicate with her mother, and Peg discovers new competence in parenting. The situation for Vicky is more complicated. If changes in her position in other social systems do not compensate for her separation from her mother, her new patterns may become dysfunctional.

M: Could that be why you began to disguise yourself as a thirty-year-old?

VICKY (laughing): It could, but I don't know. I just didn't notice it.

M: Trying to prove to yourself that you are taller and bigger, so you won't be left out? It can be an interesting thing. What do you do when you see Mom looking at Natalie, but not at you? What do you do to attract her attention?

VICKY: Move closer to Natalie and try to listen in (laughs). If I really wanted to get her, I could yell "Mom!" Or I could walk over and see what they're doing, and put my head close to Mom.

Vicky is trying to find a place in the new family shape by playing at being an adult. I must try to find out what her position in the previous family was. If she was in a central position before, or closer to her father, this new family organization may become very difficult for her. Fortunately, it appears that her position in the trio is similar to her position in the previous family.

M: How was it when Mom was married to Dad? Were you closer to Dad?

VICKY: I think we were the same.

M: There are always differences. Let me ask Natalie. Who was closer to Dad?

NATALIE: I think I was.

M: And when Dad left, did you become closer to Mom?

NATALIE: Yes, but I think Vicky did too.

MOTHER: I think I've become closer to both of them. Maybe Natalie more than Vicky, but I think both of them are . . .

M: That's not the way Vicky experiences it.

MOTHER: Is that true, Vicky?

VICKY: I'm . . . like . . . closer to you than I was before. But just a little. Natalie's a lot more, and you go to her more than you do to me.

Some tasks change for the divorced adult, notably spouse functioning and the relationships with peers. But the single parent must continue fulfilling the socializing tasks of parenting, though both the experience and the execution of those tasks change.

M: Who was the person in your marriage who did the disciplining?

MOTHER: I think I was.

NATALIE: No, it was Daddy.

MOTHER: That's interesting.

M: See, people have different experiences. What happened since Daddy left?

NATALIE: She does the disciplining.

VICKY: Yes.

M: Did she get tougher?

VICKY: No.

NATALIE: Easier.

VICKY: My dad always horned in on our fights. Mom didn't have a chance to handle it.

NATALIE: And now that my dad's not there to horn in or anything, she does it by herself. And she's not as hard as my dad was.

M: Is she tougher than she was before?

VICKY: I think she changed. She's not as tough, because she can understand what we're fighting about.

M: That's kind of curious. I would expect she'd be stricter now that she has to do it all.

NATALIE: She didn't want to be that strict with us before. But since my dad had control of everyone, she just went along with him even when she didn't want to. When he left, she was on her own to do whatever she wanted.

Parents necessarily observe children from the perspective of their own life experience. When there are two parents, there are always two points of view. This stereoscopic view may produce a calibration of two sight lines that corrects for error, but of course it also introduces the possibility of carrying differences and conflicts from the spouse field over into the parenting areas. Vicky and Natalie experience the mother's parenting now as a response to their behavior, not to her conflictual relationship with her husband.

M: That's an interesting idea. How do you explain that?

VICKY: Well, if we're fighting she'll yell at us. And most of the time then, we talk it out and find out what it was. She's more understanding about our problems than before.

M: Are you having more fights now? Or fewer?

VICKY: I think we're having more.

M: How do you explain that?

VICKY: I think we're both getting older, and we want to share things like clothes, hairbrushes, toys—things like that. And we fight over it.

Vicky gives a developmental explanation for the sisters' increased overt conflict, but it could also be attributed to the change in the mother's style of discipline. If less control means that the children must negotiate issues directly, the increase in fighting must be seen as a positive change. It will facilitate the children's experience of negotiation and conflict resolution instead of repression.

M: And do you get the same things as Natalie?

VICKY: Sometimes. Not all the time.

M: Does Mom have different rules for Natalie?

VICKY: She can do some things that I can't because she's older.

M: What kind of things?

VICKY: Stay up later—things like that. Going out with her friends later—she's always sleeping over at Elizabeth's house.

M: And you don't like that?

VICKY: No.

M: Peg, it's clear that Vicky is experiencing difficulties with the change. Can you talk with her about that?

MOTHER: You don't like the fact that Natalie is treated differently sometimes?

VICKY: You talk to her more than you do me. It's mainly that. She has more things she's allowed to do, and you give her more privileges because she's older. I don't like that.

MOTHER: It bothers me that you think I talk to her more and I include her more than I do you. That bothers me.

M: Because it's not true? Or because it's true?

MOTHER: I'm not sure. No, it bothers me because it's probably true at times, and I don't want to do that. I want to include you in family discussions, Vicky, and fun times—you know, no matter what it is. It bothers me that I leave you out because I don't want it to be like that. I don't know what I can do. I guess maybe I have to become more aware that that's happening, so that I can include you.

M: I think if you don't do that, Peg, pretty soon you will have Vicky looking older than you. She doesn't look like a mature ten-year-old now—she's a little old lady.

MOTHER: Well, she's been telling me that she's afraid I'm going to leave her. So we've talked about that. Vicky, why are you afraid I'm going to leave you?

VICKY: Because Daddy left us.

MOTHER: Am I somehow giving you the message that I'm going to leave you?

VICKY: No. Well, sometimes.

MOTHER: Well, how?

NATALIE: Like when you go places with Mike, and when you spend more time with him. Things like that.

MOTHER: In other words, if I go out with Mike without you girls, you're afraid I won't come back?

We have seen that Vicky's sense of displacement in the family is related to the mother's and Natalie's increased closeness. But open expression of the threat occurs mostly around the relationship of Peg and Mike. Perhaps Mike's entrance into the trio when the new shape has not yet found a new balance has exacerbated the stresses inherent in transitional periods. But focusing on the threat would be a mistake, since it would detract from the developing trio's exploration and renegotiation. The mother should be able to explore her relationship with men as well as develop a new relationship with her daughters.

M: It's probably clear that she prefers to be alone with him sometimes. What do you say, Peg? Vicky is afraid you're going to abandon her.

MOTHER: I say it's not true. My love for Mike is different from the love I have for you and Natalie. You know that! You can't be that dumb. (*All laugh.*)

VICKY: I know she won't leave us. But sometimes, most of the time, I just get the feeling that she might.

M: Aren't kids marvelous, Peg? The way they make parents feel guilty?

MOTHER: Why do you think they do that? Not them, particularly, but children?

M: Because they're mean. (*All laugh.*) Don't you know that?

MOTHER: Selfish?

M: Of course. What do you think about that, girls?

NATALIE: Me or her (*laughs*)?

M: Both.

NATALIE: I guess we are pretty selfish because we don't want to share her with anybody else. Not Mike or anybody.

M: When Dad was in the family, didn't you also think about not wanting to share Dad with Mom or Mom with Dad?

NATALIE: No, because he was part of the family. He was my father. But Mike's not.

M: So you feel he's an intruder. Do you spill coffee on his shirt?

I begin, in a light banter, to encourage the exploration and verbalization of fantasies of aggression.

MOTHER: What kind of things do you do?
NATALIE: Nothing, really.
M: Does he smoke? You could burn a hole in his pocket. Does he talk with you at all? Or is he an exclusive friend of your mom's, the way Elizabeth is your exclusive friend?
NATALIE: He talks about fun things, like going skiing—things like that. Not really important things.
M: What kind of things would you like to talk to him about?
NATALIE: Nothing, really. I just feel uncomfortable talking. I mean, I don't mind if I just talk to him, but about important things I would feel a little bit uncomfortable.

Proximity between a child and her parent's new companion can be stressful for the child. Sometimes single parents push children and the new companion into a premature and uncomfortable relationship.

M: Does your father have a girlfriend? (*They nod.*) How do you feel about that?
NATALIE: Well, it's not bad because she's a lot younger than he is. She's only twelve years older than me. So I feel like she's my girlfriend. She likes the same things I do. We're alike. Mike and I aren't alike.
M: What about you, Vicky?
VICKY: I . . . we don't live with our dad, so it seems different. When we go up there to see him, we spend most of the time at his apartment. She comes over only sometimes.

If the girls lived with their father, the father's girlfriend might well be seen as an intruder, but Mike would be "all right."

M: But Mike is really a threat?
VICKY: Yes.
M: Well, between the two of you, maybe you can really scare him away. Then you'll have Mom to yourself.

They all laughed, and the girls set out to reassure Peg. The session finished in a light mood, and the Jansons left as they had arrived—correctly considering themselves a normal family, managing to keep life's stresses within a manageable range. The interview had, however, highlighted certain areas of concern. Vicky's ersatz maturity was particularly worrisome. Would she find a way of growing down to her ten years of age? Or more precisely, would the development of the trio offer its members new possibilities? Would the Mother/Natalie dyad offer space to Vicky? Would Natalie's position as her mother's confidante trap her into that role, which can be as constricting as any deviant position? Would Peg find the freedom to explore adult companionship without feeling that she was betraying her daughters?

I saw the Jansons again eighteen months after the first interview, two years after the father's departure. In the following transcript, interview segments have been organized to highlight the changes that had occurred in the intervening months.

M: I'm interested in what has happened in the last year and a half. How are things with you?

MOTHER: Well, I think basically we're doing much better. I think last time we saw you, we were in the process of moving.

M: That was a major event. Tell me what happened.

MOTHER: Very major, a big step. But we made it. It was very trying; it was almost as bad as the separation because it was a physical change and an emotional change. We had to move away from our friends, and a neighborhood we were used to, and I think we were all fearful about it. When we moved, Vicky had a lot of trouble at school. She got into a class that wasn't right for her—it was horrible, wasn't it, Vicky? Of course it affected us at home, and I had to get a child study team and have her evaluated. I didn't get much help from the principal; in fact, I got a big runaround.

M: What happened, Vicky?

VICKY: Well, my teacher would assign things that she didn't know how to do herself. Stuff like that. And the kids there are different from where I used to live. Some of the kids—not all of them—don't have any upbringing. Most of my friends were like me. They had upbringing.

M: Let me understand what it means to be "like you." What does it mean to be like them? Can you describe them?

VICKY: They were rude. Most of them were ignorant.

NATALIE: Tell him what happened.

MOTHER: An example, or an event that happened.

VICKY: For instance, if someone is talking and another person says shut up, they'll start punching, because . . .

MOTHER: If I may interrupt, there was no structure in the classroom. There was no control. And I know that Vicky needs definite rules. She needs to know what is expected of her and what the consequences are if she doesn't measure up. And there was none of that. If she didn't perform, nothing happened. If she did perform, then that was okay too. Because—but tell Dr. Minuchin how it's different this year.

VICKY: Well, this year I have a new teacher. He takes more control over the class. If you hand in your homework, you get a higher grade than someone who didn't hand it in. And if you goof around you get in trouble.

M: Do you have many friends this year, or . . .

NATALIE: Yes, she does!

MOTHER: You think she has a lot of girlfriends?

NATALIE: Yeah! I get sick of answering the phone.

It seems the Jansons moved a notch down on the socioeconomic scale when they changed neighborhoods. Vicky found herself in a more complex and heterogeneous classroom than she was used to. But she seems to have managed the transition successfully after initial difficulties, with the help of Natalie and her mother. In this transaction we have also seen the mother's delegation of executive functions to Natalie. This process, which occurs in many families in transition, can be helpful to the mother and valuable for Natalie, allowing her to experiment with adult functions. The effect on Vicky will depend on the flexibility of the new family's organizations in other contexts. I begin to explore other family transactions to clarify this issue.

M: Vicky, how is your sister treating you?

VICKY: She's the same as she was before. We get in fights sometimes.

M: Does she still think she has to help you because you're not grown-up?

VICKY: I don't think she wants me to grow up.

M: What does she do that makes you think that?

VICKY: Well, if I wear something of hers, or I get something new, sometimes she'll criticize it, or say "You look too old in that."

NATALIE: The only time I say that is when you try to wear my shoes.

VICKY: I don't wear your shoes.

NATALIE: You like to wear my boots.

VICKY: Boy! That one day, just because I wanted to . . .

M: So you think she treats you as if you're younger?

VICKY: No, she treats me as if she doesn't want me to get any older.

NATALIE: Well, I don't feel that way at all.

VICKY: You used to.

NATALIE: Yes, last year. But I don't feel that way any more.

VICKY: Well, but when we get in a fight you act . . .

NATALIE: Like . . . ?

VICKY: You tell me what to do. But other times you talk to me about things that go on in school. (*To Minuchin.*) She tells me things she does. Things she doesn't even tell Mom.

M: Okay. That's a big change.

It seems that although Natalie acts as a parental child, the relationship between the siblings is fluid. Bickering and competition alternate with periods of sharing, confidence, and cooperation. This flexibility in their transactions is a good indicator of a healthy family organization.

M: Vicky, one of the things I remember your telling me is that after the separation you were feeling quite at a loss. Your mom and your sister were close, and you felt left out. Are they still pals? Are you still left out?

VICKY: No, not really. My mom and I are basically friends. Once in a while she and Natalie will talk about something they don't want me to hear, but usually I'm included. And sometimes I talk to my mom, and I don't want Natalie to know.

M: Who changed that?

VICKY: I guess my mom and I both. We just tried to get closer.

M: How did that happen? Did your mom try to make space for you? Or did you get pushy and demand more space?

VICKY: Both, I guess.

MOTHER: I see it that way too. I think once I became aware of Vicky's concerns, I was more sensitive to the fact that she felt left out. And Vicky did push for more, to have more of me. I became more aware and sensitive to that and made room for her, I guess.

M: Natalie, what happened in that process?

NATALIE: I didn't do anything. They just did it.

M: But you noticed that it was happening?

NATALIE: Yeah.

M: Did Mom talk with you and tell you about it?

NATALIE: No.

M: Okay. How would you say the situation is now? Is your mom still kind of closer to you?

NATALIE: Yeah.

M: And Vicky?

NATALIE: Well, she's friends with my mom too.

In the first interview Vicky's position in the family seemed deviant, and her attempts to find a solution through ersatz maturity seemed doomed to failure. A year and a half ago Vicky was trying to solve an interpersonal problem through maneuvers of denial— "I don't need you; I'm an adult." Now it is clear that Vicky's exploration was only one of the many experiments with change that occur in transitional situations. Her present position in the trio seems functional.

M: Mike was almost part of the family a year ago. Is he still around?

NATALIE: Yeah.

M: So he's a permanent fixture now. Does he live with you?

MOTHER: He has his own home.

M: What's your relationship with him, Natalie?

NATALIE: Oh, we talk sometimes. I'm not friends with him, but I talk to him on the phone.

M: About what?

NATALIE: How are you, how's work, how's school. Just conversation.

M: A year and a half ago you described Mike as Mom's friend, but nothing to you.

NATALIE: It's a little better.

M: Do you think they'll get married?

NATALIE: No. She doesn't want to get married.

M: Would you like Mike to join the family?

NATALIE: Not really.

M: Why? What would happen to the family situation?

NATALIE: It would be different.

M: How?

NATALIE: Just different. He'd probably take up more of my mom's time. And I'd have to relate to him more probably.

M: And you don't want to?

NATALIE: No. Well, I do, but I don't.

It appears that the Mike/Natalie relationship has not changed. Natalie still sees him as an intruder on the trio's territory, and a possible threat to her relationship with her mother.

M: Vicky, what about you? What's your feeling?

VICKY: Oh, I don't know. We talk sometimes when he's over. We talk more like friends. I guess I have a better friendship with him than last time.

M: That's interesting. You've become closer to him?

VICKY: A little.

M: How did that happen?

VICKY: He acts friendly toward me and Natalie. But usually Natalie is with her friends or doing something, and I'm usually home.

M: So she's the one who pushes him out?

VICKY: No, she doesn't push him out. She's just out of the way when he comes over.

MOTHER: I disagree.

M: Talk with Natalie about that.

MOTHER: I think you have a way of letting him know, very subtly, that you're . . . it's "Don't get too close to me."

M: But Vicky has accepted him?

MOTHER: I think so.

NATALIE: I accept him. I just don't like him too much.

MOTHER: Okay. Vicky's more accepting, more friendly.

M: Do you go out with Mike and Vicky sometimes?

MOTHER: Yes. But I don't think it's any more than with Mike and Natalie.

NATALIE: I do. Of course I'm never home.

MOTHER: That's true. Natalie is pulling away to build her own life. You know she has her activities and her friends, and they all go to a dance or a date or a party. More so than Vicky. That time we all went skiing, where were you?

NATALIE: I was babysitting.

MOTHER: We'd already made plans, so we went without her. Another time we were going on a trip she had basketball practice and didn't want to miss it. So again it was Vicky and Mike and me. So many times Natalie has her own agenda. She has the choice of doing what we're doing or doing her own thing.

M: And you prefer to go along, Vicky?

VICKY: Yes.

Clearly Vicky's position changes in the context of the quartet. When her parents separated, she was the only family member whose losses were not immediately balanced by new possibilities. In her depression, she fantasized herself as self-sufficient (at the age of ten). Mike's entrance into the family opened up for her the possibility of proximity to the mother and Mike as a member of a new trio. Natalie continues to respond to Mike's position in the family by accelerating her adolescent push for autonomy.

M: Does Mike have other children?

MOTHER: He has a fifteen-year-old son.

M: What's your relationship with him?

NATALIE: I talk to him, but we're not really friendly, I guess. I mean, I don't act cruel.

M: You just don't like him.

NATALIE: Not really.

M: I like that. You're straight. What about you, Vicky? Do you like him?

VICKY: We're friendly, but not close friends.

MOTHER: Vicky's closer to Mike's son than Natalie is. They seem to get along better.

VICKY: If we go on a trip and Natalie's not there, we may hang around together.

NATALIE: I went skiing.

VICKY: Yeah, but you can't ski.

NATALIE: I ski as well as you do!

M: What is Mike's feeling about your children?

MOTHER: I think he likes them very much. He accepts them.

M: Does he feel the distance?

MOTHER: Oh yes. He told me that he feels closer to Vicky than he does to Natalie, and he senses that Vicky feels closer to him than Natalie does.

The family's expansion to include Mike's child has allowed Vicky to explore proximity with an older "sibling" in a position closer to her own. But this has also introduced new stresses in the Vicky/Natalie relationship.

M: Okay. There was another family—your father and his girl-friend.

NATALIE: They're going to get married.

M: Is it the same girlfriend?

NATALIE: Yes.

M: What happened there? Last time you seemed to have an easier relationship with her than with Mike.

NATALIE: I'm still closer to her than Mike.

VICKY: I'm not.

M: Okay. That's nice, very nice, because you were a little bit of a copycat before, and you've changed. What happened in your relationship with your father?

NATALIE: We got closer.

M: In what way?

NATALIE: He talks to me more now, more about personal things, just everything, really.

M: He talks to you about his girlfriend?

NATALIE: Sometimes. Mostly work. Or my mom, or Vicky.

M: He talks with you about Vicky?

NATALIE: Yeah. If we get in a fight, or my mom and I get in a fight.

M: Can you tell me more about these talks?

NATALIE: Well, when my mom and he were going to go to court, he would talk to me about it. One night—Vicky, you weren't home . . .

VICKY: He talked to me the next day.

NATALIE: Right. The next day he talked to you, but that was different. He talked differently to me than he did to you.

M: What do you mean by that?

NATALIE: Well, he just told her what was going on, but he told me how he felt about it. He was—like, getting out all his frustrations.

MOTHER: And he didn't do that with Vicky?

VICKY: No.

M: That means he treats you more as a person in whom he can confide.

NATALIE: Yes.

The relationship between the father and his daughters seems to have followed developmental lines. Natalie, the adolescent, has become the father's confidante and liaison with the old family. Vicky has tried unsuccessfully to compete, but, as we have seen, she is also developing a closer relationship with her mother and Mike.

In the transition after a divorce, the parents must negotiate how to continue parenting when they are no longer spouses. This inevitably brings forth the need to agree about finances. In the Janson family this area was managed uneventfully until the father decided to marry again. The mother, deciding she had been exploited, requested increased child support, possibly because her ex-husband's decision to marry again temporarily reawakened old demands for loyalty.

MOTHER: We couldn't get together on it, so my lawyer went to court. The children were very fearful because my ex said something about fighting it and that I might wind up getting less.

BOTH GIRLS: Yeah.

MOTHER: And he said that he was such a nice guy that even if the judge reduced it, he would still pay the same. I was upset about the whole thing because I think he used the two of them to get to me.

NATALIE: You make it sound like he was brainwashing us!

MOTHER: No, my perception was that he was using you both in this instance. That's how it came across.

M: Would you say he wanted both of you to think he was right?

NATALIE: Yes. He was just explaining it. I told him what my mom said.

M: And you think that you were right, Peg?

MOTHER: Yes.

NATALIE: Then you were using us too. You were saying you were right, and he was saying he was right.

MOTHER: I didn't ask you to tell him.

NATALIE: Well, he didn't ask us to tell you!

MOTHER: Did I say anything to you to make you afraid?

NATALIE: No . . . well, what would you say? "I'm not going to take his money any more?"

M: She could say she wouldn't let you go see him.

NATALIE: She wouldn't say that.

M: Oh, but she could.

MOTHER: I could have. I could have retaliated. I explained the facts to you, that's all.

NATALIE: He said he explained the facts too.

M: What happened in the end?

NATALIE: It stayed the same.

MOTHER: The judge didn't increase or decrease it.

M: Okay. In that fight, whose side were you on?

NATALIE: My dad's.

M: Vicky?

VICKY: My dad's.

M: That's fascinating.

MOTHER: It certainly is! Especially when they want more and more things all the time, and I have to tell them I don't have the money.

M: From a financial point of view, you should have been on your mother's side.

MOTHER: Right. I think he got to you and tried to make you feel sorry for him.

NATALIE: He didn't.

MOTHER: That's the way it came across to me.

VICKY: You weren't there.

MOTHER: Well, that's how it came across from the way you two talked. Mostly you, Vicky. The way you talked to me. You said something like "You want everything from him, and he's not going to have anything."

VICKY: I didn't say that.

While the girls are in different camps in relation to the new family, they are both loyal to their father. They felt that their mother's challenge was unjustified. After all her work for the girls, Peg is surprised and feels betrayed. But it is an indication of good parenting that the girls could rally to their father and feel free to express their views without fearing that this would endanger their relationship with their mother.

M: Have there been changes in your mother?

VICKY: Since last time? She's changed.

M: In what way?

NATALIE: She's nicer.

VICKY: She does more things.

M: That's a big change. Since the divorce she's become more active. Why is that?

VICKY: I don't know.

M: Was your father sitting on her? How did that happen?

VICKY: I don't know. I guess Mike is more active.

M: So that means that a change in your mom has been brought about by Mike.

NATALIE: She's more of her own person now.

M: How so?

NATALIE: Well, she's not Dan's wife. She's Peg.

M: But she could be Mike's girlfriend.

NATALIE: She acts more like herself at home.

M: Explain that. This is very interesting. Explain so I can understand.

NATALIE: She's not as crabby. She's not as strict.

MOTHER: With rules? Around the house, you mean?

NATALIE: Yes. You're not as old-fashioned.

MOTHER: My ex-husband was very rigid about a lot of things. So I guess I ran the house . . .

NATALIE: For him.

MOTHER: He wanted to have meals at a certain time, schedules—that kind of thing. Now we're a lot more flexible. If you want to eat in front of the TV set, you can. If they want to have sandwiches for dinner, that's okay.

M: You said she's her own person. That's a catchy phrase. What does it mean?

NATALIE: She just acts different. She acts the way she wants to act, not the way she thinks my dad wants her to act. She acts like herself. Before, she used to act like my dad.

M: Now how has your dad changed? Did he change?

NATALIE: Yeah.

VICKY: He's not as old-fashioned. Not as straight. Not as crabby.

M: So you think your dad went through some of the same changes as your mom?

NATALIE: The only thing is that he's not real active.

MOTHER: Is he as rigid as he used to be?

NATALIE: No.

MOTHER: You know, you had to straighten the magazine piles when he was around.

VICKY: Not now.

M: Why is that?

NATALIE: I think it's his girlfriend. She's younger, and she acts younger.

VICKY: She's more into new things. New styles.

M: You know, you could be a commercial for divorce.

MOTHER: Get divorced and be a new person!

M: Yes, that's a fascinating thing. Is that what you think?

VICKY: In this case.

The rejection of the previous family together with a focus on the opportunities brought by change seem to have created a model of individual growth in dismemberment. If so, Natalie, Vicky, and thousands of other children of divorce hold ideas clearly different from my generation's focus on individual growth through conflict resolution. Perhaps the most positive model would preserve the memory of good elements from the previous

family, while incorporating the concept of differences in the new
one.

M: You're saying that both your father and your mother have
changed since they separated. What about your feelings, Peg?
Your daughters paint a very interesting picture.

MOTHER: I can't speak for him, but I know I've changed.

M: In what way?

MOTHER: I feel more—I hate to use the same phrase—more my
own person. I make my own decisions. I don't have to confer
with anyone. I don't have to compromise. If I want to do something a certain way, or if I don't want to do something, I don't
have to.

M: Vicky attributes this change to Mike. Is that true?

MOTHER: I think he's acted as a catalyst. There are things I would
have liked to do while I was married, but Dan wasn't really en-
thusiastic about it. I wanted to try skiing. He always had some
excuse not to. I wanted us to play tennis together. No, he didn't
want to do that.

NATALIE: You played tennis together.

MOTHER: Once or twice. There was usually an excuse for him not
to do it with me. He was into accumulating material possessions more than doing things.

NATALIE: Yes. And now that you don't have those material things,
it's "Oh God I wish I had this, or I wish I had that."

MOTHER: Oh sure. People are never satisfied.

Natalie keeps the father's "ghost voice" in the family. She
doesn't want her mother to forget.

M: Tell me, why don't you want to marry Mike? Does Mike want
to marry you?

MOTHER: No. But he'd like it if we lived together and merged our
lives somehow into a more permanent relationship.

M: And you don't want that?

MOTHER: I would like to merge our relationship and make it more
permanent. And he would too. We're having trouble with our
own insecurities, getting it together. I'd like him to move into
my house so I don't have to move again with the two children.

He doesn't want to do that; he wants me to move into his house. I guess I don't want to do that because I don't feel too secure about moving again. I know what a tremendous burden it was. We use all these excuses, and they really are excuses: my house is bigger, my house is closer, he says his mortgage is lower, his neighborhood is nicer—it's all crap, is what it is. The bottom line is that we're both scared. We recognize that, and we've also recognized that right now we're at a stalemate in what we're going to do.

M: But you've been together for three years now.

MOTHER: Two and a half.

M: And you would like to make it a foursome if conditions were okay. If he accepted your conditions—

MOTHER: And he would like to do it if I accepted his conditions.

M: You want him to come join you.

MOTHER: Right now I really think it's a power struggle on his part.

M: You think you would accept him if Mom said so, Natalie?

NATALIE: I don't care either way.

M: Tell me, now that your father is going to be married, has he suggested that you live with him?

NATALIE: He didn't offer. But when he talked about child support, he said if I want to come and live with him, I can. He said he didn't ever want me to use it as a threat, though. No "I'm going to go live with Daddy."

M: What about you, Vicky?

VICKY: Same thing.

M: That means this is an option for you, at some point. Do you discuss these things with them, Peg?

MOTHER: Not with my ex-husband. I talk to the girls about it.

M: What's your opinion?

MOTHER: It's an option for them, but I think it's something they should consider very seriously. It's not like going on vacation. It's moving again, a whole new environment, a different set of rules.

VICKY: I think if he moved close by so I could go to the same school and have the same friends, I would go live with him.

M: So this is one of the things that happen when you have two parents in different territories. You can decide to live in one style of life or a different one. Have you ever threatened your mom by saying you'd go live with your dad?

NATALIE: Vicky asks me, "Why don't you go live with Daddy?"

VICKY: No! When we get in fights, you're the one who says, "I think I'm going to go live with Daddy."

Still in transition, the Jansons' family pattern is growing and changing. None of the transitional structures is inherently wrong; they are all experiments in living.

Natalie may decide to move in with her father after he remarries. Then the changed shapes will again enter into crisis, search through trial, error, and accommodation, and reach some resolution that is viable and (with luck) encouraging of growth. Mike may join the trio. He will then have to find a path to Natalie's respect and affection, while the mother feels out the appropriate distance for supporting both of them in this learning. Vicky may be helpful in the process, since she has already begun the process of gluing Mike to the trio. Perhaps. All we know for sure is that each scenario is an experiment in living. Thus, by definition, it will be carried out in an unstable field, full of visible and hidden traps. The only certainty is that there will be errors and, because of them, conflict, solutions, and growth.

Answers are born in the way we pose questions. When we look seriously at people interacting with each other, measuring their interactions and applying prevalent norms to the interpretation of our findings, our results can elicit either concern or laughter. Looking at life, as I do, as sets of unfilled promises, I think on the whole that I prefer laughter.

Most of the studies on divorce and children of divorce seem to lean more to concern. There have been many such studies published recently—in 1981, the year I first interviewed the Jansons, the United States divorce rate hit a record 1.21 million. Natalie and Vicky were two of an estimated 1.18 million children involved in divorces that year.

With the divorce rate approaching one in every two marriages, the "death of the American family" hit the headlines. And although statistically divorce seemed to be becoming a norm, almost all discussions insisted on framing it as a failure of the nuclear family. Descriptions were steeped in the language of trouble—confusion, anxiety, fear, depression, anger, and guilt. From Francke's *Growing Up Divorced:*

> Even after two years, twelve-year-old Sophie still hasn't forgiven her mother for leaving her idolized father for another man . . . "I try to get even" says the beautiful preteen . . . "I want to make my mother feel bad. I resent her. No matter what she says, I say the opposite. I want her to feel guilty. I want revenge . . ." Sophie is so used to her anger that her voice is completely matter-of-fact.

Wallerstein and Kelly, respected clinician-researchers, state in *Surviving the Breakup:* "Whatever its shortcomings the family is perceived by the child at this time as having provided the support and protection he needs. The divorce signifies the collapse of this structure and he feels alone and frightened."

If I had asked the members of the trio questions designed to elicit confusion, anxiety, fear, depression, anger, and guilt, I would have found them. But in interviewing the Jansons I played down negative emotions. When the girls showed fear of abandonment, anger at their parents, conflicts, and neurotic attempts at problem solving, I hesitated, acknowledged these as real things, smiled, and asked for a new look, a different perspective. It's not that I fail to see what other experts see. I simply prefer another framing.

My experience in family psychiatry has given me, along with a deep respect for families and their ability to support and nurture, an acceptance of their varying shapes. I accept that families will divorce and that the divorced family is a viable family organization, one of many our culture has institutionalized.

An historical and contextual perception of family change would do much to lessen the hysteria of concern over the current health of the American family. For example, consider the British family of two centuries ago. According to the sociologist Lawrence Stone, this would not have been the nuclear unit but the kin unit (the open lineage system). Stone points out that, well into the seventeenth century, marriage was largely an arrangement for the combination of properties and the continuation of family lines. The rearing of the children born to the union and the mutual support of the spouses—two of the tasks we consider to be primary functions of the nuclear family unit—were much more the business of the kin system. Relatively little importance was attached to the spouse unit. If a husband and wife grew to care for each other, there was certainly no harm done, but if mutual affection did not develop, no one considered the marriage a failure on that account. Children were commonly reared away from their parents, by wet nurses. All individuals were interchangeable. Particularly for children, the mortality rate was high. Medieval parents often gave several of their children the same name, in the hope that at least one might live to bear it into adulthood. Until the level of infant and child mortality began to decline toward the beginning of the modern age, it was simply not safe to love a baby or any individual. The family was impermanent.

With the Industrial Revolution came improved hygiene and medical care; spouses and children could survive longer. English society began to change, and so did family norms. By the mid-eighteenth century the nuclear family was the accepted ideal of the middle classes. Then for the first time the interdependence of the spouses and the rearing of children became major tasks for the nuclear unit. Stone estimates that this change in family norm took about two hundred years. In our own time family change—like everything else—is happening faster.

I can identify several different norms within my own experience. My paternal grandfather's world was solidly patriarchal. He overshadowed my grandmother and held the fear and loyalty of all ten of his children. Of course he demanded more from his sons and grandsons than from the women of the family. As the eldest boy in my family of origin, I was given the most responsibility, obligations, and respect. My siblings and I will always carry the imprint of functions strictly differentiated according to gender. But I married into another culture, in another time. My wife is a psychologist. She and my daughter "raised my consciousness" about women. Not incidentally, I learned to cook and wash dishes on the nights my wife taught. My son and daughter were raised in a more "androgynous" way (this being the unfortunate word chosen by psychologists to denote the alternation of functions at one time locked into a particular gender).

At this point in history, most Americans still think of the nuclear family as the norm—which automatically makes us think of other shapes as "incorrect." But history moves on. It seems to me that, instead of hanging ourselves up on the "normalcy" of the intact nuclear family, we should recognize change as inevitable, even normal, and set ourselves the tasks of helping families over transitional periods.

In cases of divorce, then, we would not counsel each individual family member to alleviate the pain of the breakup; we would offer instead family counseling that focuses on the creative possibilities of the new organism. Instead of creating an adversarial relationship through our legal system, we would offer family mediation. Perhaps we might even derive some forms of *rite du passage* that would join new family segments in a ritual of acceptance and healing. Divorced spouses would be expected to accept their past experiences as valid and to see the present divorced configuration as a necessary, agreed-on distancing that still supports a friendly cooperative involvement in parenting.

These vistas will seem impossible for most divorcing families today because we are still organized to defend the nuclear family. Courts and lawyers still support the adversary system; we still have the need to be loyal to only one segment of our friends. Divorce is still called a "broken home." But families are changing as society changes. In time, our institutions will catch up.

READER: Others insist on highlighting the negative aspects of divorce. You insist on highlighting its possibilities. A bias is a bias is a bias.

AUTHOR: Touché. I would like to repeat, however, that from a historical perspective what we're seeing is just another blip in the curves of family change. It is not necessary either to support or to oppose a process that will continue despite our preferences.

READER: Maybe family breakup is a good thing. I read a book by David Cooper, *The Death of the Family*, which said families are conservative molds that rob family members of their individuality.

AUTHOR: That was true in the sixties.

READER: But you claim that families further individual growth.

AUTHOR: That was also true in the sixties.

READER: But they're different questions! You're giving the same answer.

AUTHOR (*smiling*): That too was true in the sixties.

READER: I thought that joke was very funny—the first time I heard it. If you can be serious for a moment, let me ask you something. If I understand the design of your book, you are trying to challenge established views about the family and also help me to see my own reality differently. Right?

AUTHOR: Yes. I want to challenge the precise separation of context and people.

READER: Well, the trio is the clinical description of a particular family. It's a nice case, but it's merely anecdotal. Stone's material sounds interesting, but—

AUTHOR: Let me tell you a fable.

READER: Is it relevant to my question?

AUTHOR: I think so. Pretend that one day I told the Jansons' story to a beaver. As usual, she was building a dam.

"I liked the divorce story," the beaver said, adding a small branch to the dam.

"Yes. It has to do with man's idea of time and how things are done," said the pond (who, as you know, has been studying Man since Narcissus).

"Anything unusual about that?" The beaver added another twig.

"Man is surprised when things balance out. Humans don't know how to build a dam."

"But everyone knows it's a matter of forces and counterforces, levels and balances," proclaimed the beaver in a display of scientific erudition.

"Not everyone. Humans think everyone builds his dam alone."

"That's stupid!" The beaver patted mud into the twigs.

"It is indeed." The pond made a new detour, and laughed.

"I don't understand a word you're saying," the therapist complained.

"That's because you spend your time describing deviancy," the pond replied severely.

"What is deviancy?" the beaver asked.

"It's the name people give to pain."

"Why do they change the names of things? It's stupid! Things remain the same."

"Oh no," said the pond. "Through magic incantations the named lose their own shape, and become more and more what they're called."

"That's strange," said the beaver, diving into a tunnel.

"Yes, it is," the pond replied, beginning to play with the breeze.

READER: I don't see how this fable relates to system or to divorce!
AUTHOR: Oh. Well, it's a nice fable anyway.

Quartet

Patterns of Remarriage

This chapter was written with Virginia Goldner.

"Hi," the new neighbor introduces himself. "I'm Leonard Knox. This is my wife, Helen Leopold, and our kids Terry Coburn and Glen Fisher." This blended "yours, mine, and ours" family shape is a testimony to the flexibility and strength of human beings, for it can become extraordinarily complex. Even within the new nuclear unit, problems abound. The spouses' new life develops under the critical eye of children whose view of the couple is organized by their experience in the previous family group. Each parent must respond to his or her own children, who usually need protection in the beginning period, as well as pay special attention to the process of getting to know the stepchildren. At the same time, it may be necessary to adjust to the estranged parents' emotional responses. The slow accommodation process necessary for the development of a new couple collides with the necessity to function from the beginning as a parental team. The children have been coopted into a new organism not of their making. They must distance themselves from one parent, accommodate to the new stepparent, and make friends with their ready-made siblings, frequently in a different geographical space—new home, new schools, new friends.

The new problems may seem like the product of a deviant and mischievous computer, testing the ingenuity of humanity's adaptation to social constructs. For the most part, though, it works out. At once there is a new pattern, already developing and changing.

The Smiths came for therapy because Matt, now sixteen, was having difficulties in school. A brilliant student up to a year ago, he was not studying and annoyed teachers and peers by endless polemics in which his demand for precision in language sometimes took on bizarre characteristics. At home he engaged both parents in tests of power and independence. One could think of a typical acute outburst of adolescence, except that at times his language became incomprehensible. This frightened the parents, and the father's concern and fear took the form of increasing control and a barrage of irrational yelling.

The Smiths married three years ago. Joan had been divorced for some time, living alone with her older son (who left for college six months after the marriage) and with her other son Jim, who is now eighteen. Steven married Joan one month after his divorce became final. His son Matt came to live with him and Joan; his two other children remained with his first wife. Steven is a successful businessman. Joan is a teacher.

I saw the Smiths in eight sessions over four weeks. The excerpts of the therapy presented here are not intended to illustrate therapeutic techniques, but rather to elucidate the flexibilities and pitfalls of this family form. The fact that the family changed so rapidly in response to therapy indicates that the symptoms were the result of transitional experimentations with new forms.

After the family members defined themselves in their first session—who came with whom, how long the first marriages lasted, the separations, how old the new family is, and so on—I continued with my usual opening, a mild indirect question: "Who would like to tell me why you've come to see me?"

JOAN: Well, it has a long background, but the most recent instance was about two or three weeks ago, I guess. We were in the kitchen, and after dinner Steven told Matt that he had called the school and asked for information about Matt. And then Matt said he knew how he was doing in school, but he didn't want to tell anyone. I don't remember all the words that were said, but Matt said something and Steven tried to understand what it was that Matt was saying. And Matt was saying "That's not what I said," and it was that kind of back-and-forth thing for quite a while. Finally Steven got angry, because every time he would try to interpret something, Matt would say that wasn't what he'd said. And I didn't say anything at all. But when they started getting angry—that's why my feelings get involved, because I don't feel comfortable having that unpleasantness. It's hateful to me.

MINUCHIN: And what did you do?

JOAN: I got into it, and I guess I got very upset. I got angry, and defensive.

We see here one of the possible problems in the transitional periods of a blended family. The father/son dysfunctional interaction activates the wife, who enters to support her husband. Experiencing Steven's pain, Joan tries to help him resolve his difficulties with Matt. But by doing so, she blocks a pathway that otherwise might continue to some sort of resolution. Furthermore, Joan's entrance to get her husband off the hook is not accepted by Matt, who told me: "She is not my mother."

M: How do you remember it, Steven?

STEVEN: Pretty much the same way. When Matt was in junior high, we got all kinds of warning notices and we went to the school a couple of times to see the teachers. I wanted Matt to stop saying that it was somebody else's problem, that it was this teacher or that teacher, or some other thing. So when he got to high school this year I talked to a guidance counselor, and I asked him to come up with some kind of progress report that Matt could see before the end of the term. He told me what the teacher's reactions to Matt were, and so on. So when I got home that evening, I sat down with Matt and asked him again how he was doing. I can't remember which way the conversation went, but basically what Matt was saying to me was—first, he didn't know how he was doing, and then he did know how he was doing but he wasn't going to tell me. I guess that's what it amounted to. Then we got into . . . let's see. He didn't want to tell me because I would want him to work harder, or something like that. I kept telling him I didn't want him to work harder, I just wanted him to know how he was doing. And the thing got to a brawl; I don't know what else to call it. I got frustrated, so I started shouting. I grabbed him, I'm sure, and sat him down in a chair, and that's about the time Joan got involved in it. Because I get frustrated after a point and don't know what to do with it.

Throughout this long speech Steven has been talking at Matt, sending urgent nonverbal signals: "Listen to me, recognize that I love you, understand that I want to help you." Matt has been signaling disengagement—looking at the ceiling, shaking his head, yawning elaborately. This has increased Steven's sense of frustration, pushing him to talk longer. The father's pain and sense of impotence are as clear as the nonresolution of the end of his speech; small wonder that Joan has developed the habit of rushing to his rescue.

M: Matt, is . . .

MATT (*to Steven*): You're saying that you were yelling and I was yelling. I can see that as so. You said about how I got angry, you got angry, you got frustrated, it's true. Because it is. But what I'm trying to say is that I feel you're getting in this too much, and I feel that you're going to have to let go of some of it. And I'm not saying that you have to let go totally, but what I'm saying is that I think you're caring too much, in a sense, if you want to put it that way, because—after all, I'm trying to be more independent, but I think part of the trouble is that you have trouble realizing how I am and what I am. I've seen a lot of things happen to me, I know how my world has crumbled in the past. But I feel that I'm strong enough a person to realize what's going on, and I feel something's going to have to change. The only way to do it is to fight back. I can't see change through any other way. That's basically what I have to say.

STEVEN: Well I guess, Matt, I really don't know what your response was. Are you trying to tell us that we're supposed to leave you alone?

MATT: You said earlier that you just wanted to find out how I was doing in school. But you think I can do better in school. So that raises the question as to whether—did you really want to find out how I was doing, or did you really want to push me somewhere, or did you really want me to accept that?

Matt has prolonged his speech with long pauses and elaborate mental searchings for the right word. These pauses—a demand for equal time?—increased his father's frustration. There are three explicit and many implicit questions in Matt's last statement; their proliferation and ambiguity make any answer that will satisfy him impossible. This is the smokescreen of words Steven gets whenever he tries to reach out to his son. Concomitantly, Matt is activated by his father's indirectness and hedging.

M: Matt, you asked a question. Now find out the answer.

MATT: I asked several questions.

M: Yes. Let him answer.

STEVEN: What was the question, Matt?

MATT: Whether you wanted to push me to do more work—

STEVEN: No, I didn't.

MATT: Or whether—

STEVEN: No, I didn't. That's not what I wanted to do.

MATT: Okay. Or whether you wanted me to know what I was doing and what you were doing, or whether you wanted to—

STEVEN: You're losing me. What I . . .

MATT: I asked three questions, and the third one, I think, was whether you wanted—

STEVEN: Just a minute, Matt. Did you hear the answer to the first question?

MATT: Yeah.

STEVEN: I must be tired, Matt—I am tired. I'm not sure any more what we're talking about. I mean, I know the general subject that I'm talking about, but I don't really know what we're talking about. Are you asking me what I was trying . . .

M: Steven, can you change seats with Joan, so Joan is next to Matt? (*They change seats.*) Now, can you two talk? I want to know if this is just a difficulty with Steven. Can you continue talking, Matt?

MATT: Okay, I kind of see it as another repetition of your push to change me.

JOAN: And how about when your father told you that's not what he wants?

MATT: He wanted me to do better, and that was it. Right?

JOAN: No. He was trying to tell you that what he wanted was for you to know, so you wouldn't have any big surprises. And you didn't seem to understand that, or believe him.

MATT: Because I already knew. I already knew what I was doing, and it would be no surprise to me, obviously. It would be to you.

JOAN: But we're the ones who get called in when you have problems, so we should know. We don't like hearing it at the last minute.

All of us have experienced some variation of this complicated do-si-do. Readers who have adolescent children will find the dance all too familiar and will understand Joan and Steven's frustration and pain. Others, remembering their own adolescent struggles for autonomy, may empathize with Matt's equally understandable frustration. It is part of normal family development that its members' needs at times demand different solutions. During such periods stress, confusion, and conflict are the yeast of negotiation and growth. But for the Smiths or any other reconstituted family, the problem is even more complicated. The family is experiencing two divergent developmental periods at once. As a young family, barely three years old, they must negotiate issues of belonging, increased proximity, and cooperation. As a family with adolescent children, they must also deal with problems of autonomy and distancing. Each of these stages tries the patience and wisdom of members of any family. So it is not surprising that the Smiths have become stuck in trying to handle both at once.

I continue the session exploring the different subsystems in the family, probing for areas of expansion that might facilitate change. First, I explore the husband/wife dyad.

M: Steven, there must be ways of telling Matt that he should communicate with you in ways you can understand.

STEVEN: That's one of the big reasons I think we're trying to do this together with you. I want to learn. I had to laugh before, when you said I talk in long sentences, because I guess I really do. And if I can learn not to do that—

M: Joan will help you. Can you, Joan?

JOAN: I have.

M: You've changed him?

JOAN: When we were first married I used to argue when he would come *at* me with these long persuasive arguments.

M: And he has accommodated to you? Because a marriage is always a process of accommodation.

JOAN: I know he has. In our arguments I know I'm not as intimidated as I was when we were first married. He listens to me more, I think. I used to have to explain feelings. I used to say I was angry about something, and he used to tell me I shouldn't be or explain why I shouldn't be or give me good reasons for not having those feelings. There weren't a whole lot of problems. The most were in how to argue, that was our biggest thing.

M: In what ways have you changed to accommodate to him?

JOAN: I used to tease in ways that hurt him. I had to learn to control my tongue and not be so quick with a sharp retort. I come from a big family and we kidded that way, and I had friends who used to do the same thing. But Steven wasn't used to it and I used to hurt his feelings. I don't do that, I try not to.

M: In what other ways did Joan change?

STEVEN: The one thing I can think of right now is about arguments. We used to get into very violent arguments and it used to escalate quickly and within five or ten minutes I would hear her yelling things like "I'm going to leave, I'm going to take the kids and go." Now our arguments aren't so dramatic. We kind of talk things out more.

Traveling through life with different experiential baggage, Joan and Steven have collided, equivocated, and misinterpreted, just like any other couple learning to become a two-bodied organism. Slowly they learned to read each other and evolved a new "culture," with its own rules for developing and maintaining coexistence.

How did the children fare? Joan had been divorced for some years before her remarriage. She and her children had formed a relatively stable family form. Steven married one month after his divorce, having separated from his first wife a year earlier. Matt had lived first with his mother, then alone with his father for about six months before Steven remarried. In one year, then,

Joan's older son has left for college and Jim had begun to drift away from his mother. Matt found himself very much in the middle of the new family, caught in the turbulence of his parents' divorce and his decision to live with his father instead of his mother and two older siblings. In the new family pattern, he was also caught between two mothers and their different styles of mothering. This feeling emerges clearly as, continuing the exploration of dyads, I ask Joan and Matt to talk.

M: Joan, in what way did you change your relation to Matt, and in what way do you think Matt has changed in relation to you in these last three years?

JOAN: He's aloof. If I hug him, he won't hug me back. He doesn't want me to hug him.

M: But he's sixteen now.

JOAN: Well, I don't hug him all the time. But you know, there are occasions—I do it with all my children.

M: Matt, in what way did Joan change to accommodate to you in the last three years?

MATT: I think I've gotten more across to her where I am. I think she's trying to be too much of a mother to me, and I think that's wrong. I think she wants to be good, but that's wrong for me. Because that puts me in the middle.

M: The middle?

MATT: Between my real mother and Joan. Because of Joan's way of treating me, I'm mean to my mother.

M: You can't accept her disciplining you?

MATT: No, I can't. Why should I be in the position of having two mothers? I think it's unfair to Joan, to me, and to my mother.

JOAN: I was trying to be a parent, and I told you that.

MATT: You said you were trying to be a mother too.

JOAN: Well that's a parent. I was not trying to take your mother's place, Matt.

MATT: I know you weren't, but you said you were trying to be a mother.

JOAN: You thought I was trying to make it up to you because you didn't have a good home life when your parents were having problems?

MATT: I think you were trying too much at one time, and I think
    it was really unreasonable for you to expect so much from me.
JOAN: I didn't expect it as much at first, Matt. I was very sur-
    prised at how affectionate you were at first, but that was okay.
MATT: I may have liked you then, but I didn't like the way you
    kept trying to overpower me.
JOAN: I don't know how I was overpowering you, Matt.
MATT: By trying to be a mother to me.

In reconstructing their history together, Matt and Joan reveal
the pattern that has kept them frozen at an angry distance for so
long. Instead of allowing their rudimentary relationship as step-
mother and stepson to develop along those lines, they pushed
each other into fantasy roles that were inappropriate. Joan reports feeling "surprised" that Matt was so affectionate. Recipro-
cally, Matt remembers that Joan "overpowered" him by trying to
be his mother. With too much proximity too soon, the relationship exploded into conflict. In some way the family organization
locked them into this stalemate. What might have been a transitional phase in the development of their relationship became a
lasting problem that Matt and Joan are far too angry to work out.
We will see later how Steven participated in the maintenance of
this pattern. But here I am still involved in the exploration of
dyads, and I turn to Joan's son.

M: I also want to know, Jim, where you are in this family.
JIM: What do you mean where am I?
M: I am wondering if you have any space in the family since Matt
    is so central.
JIM: I guess so, I didn't ask them. I have school and I have sports
    after school, and a couple nights a week I leave right from
    sports to work and I work on weekends—so I'm not home a lot.
    But when I am home they have these talks at dinner, like the
    way they were talking at first, and I just don't want to be in the
    middle of it because half the time it ends up in an argument
    and I don't feel like being there when there's an argument. So
    as soon as I finish dinner I get up from the table and I either go
    out or go upstairs.

M: So you opt out.

JIM: Probably. They make a remark if I'm home for dinner two nights in a row.

M: So that's a way in which you accommodate to the family. You just take off.

JIM: Probably.

M: Is that what you prefer?

JIM: I thought about it and at times I think it's a house I live in, not a home. A home to me is where people are together and I don't think of it as a home, just a house.

M: In the last three years your relationship with your mother has worsened?

JIM: Oh yeah, it has. When they first got married things changed. I drifted, I guess. I didn't feel as close. There was a change right at the beginning because, the way Steven and Matt are used to, we changed from the very open to not very open. Like the way we used to kid, I guess. I was used to kidding around with my mom, and it just kind of changed. It couldn't quite be the same.

Where Matt got locked into a struggle with Joan, Jim got locked out because of it. The conflicts swirling around Matt (which sucked in both parents) displaced Jim. Moreover, Jim felt his mother slipping away—not only into the futile battles with Matt and Steven but into their family's pattern, which felt strange in contrast to what he was used to. Having lost both his mother and the familiar affective context of his family of origin, it is no wonder that Jim felt homeless. It is interesting that Jim's sense of abandonment and his underlying depression were not marked by the family as a problem. I don't know whether the labeling or the ignoring is preferable. However, the family had labeled Matt the problem and brought him to the attention of a therapist. And Matt has great talent for centrality, even at his own expense.

The next segment comes from an interview two weeks later. Joan had been quick to pick up my signals that she was interfering with Steven and Matt while trying to help. She and Steven were concentrating on letting Matt and his father work things out. Although there are still many difficulties, compare this interaction with the previous one.

STEVEN: I feel I need to try to work out a way that you can talk to me and I won't get upset.

MATT: If I seriously listened to you, you could alienate me more from the outer world.

STEVEN: I don't understand.

MATT: I feel that if I listen to you, it's going to make me look different from everybody else. Not just because of you but because of how I take it.

STEVEN: I don't know what you said, Matt.

MATT: Well, it's difficult for me to exactly say this, but I shut myself off because what you were saying was affecting my being with other people.

STEVEN: When you listen to me it affects how you are with everybody else?

MATT: It's just how I take what you say.

M: Are you saying that your father is so influential?

MATT: Yes.

M: That his thinking can organize your thinking?

MATT: Not organize, *dis*organize it.

M: His influence is that powerful?

MATT: I wouldn't put it in power terms.

M: I think you're saying that your father's opinion can be very influential.

STEVEN: But he doesn't want that!

M: I think Matt is saying that he's too close to you. Or that you're too close to him. But what you experience is that he's too distant.

STEVEN: Yes, I always thought that. I'm just trying to struggle with what to do about it.

MATT: I wouldn't worry about it so exactly now. I think we have to define it first.

STEVEN: I have trouble with those kinds of statements, I really do. I don't know what it is, but you'll say something like "Don't do this!" Or "If I were you I wouldn't bother about it." It just does something to me inside. It tightens me up.

M: That's good. It's very important for Matt to know that when he rejects you, you feel all tight inside.

STEVEN: Oh, very much so. You said a minute ago, Matt, that the things I say to you have a big effect on you and you don't want them to. But when you try to turn me off by saying "Leave me alone," or whatever, that really bothers me. It makes me upset, it really does.

M: Do you know what he's saying?

MATT: He's saying that when . . . when I reject him . . .

M: He suffers.

MATT: Yes. And when I accept him, *I* suffer.

Matt feels controlled by his father, who feels dismissed by Matt. Each feels the other is too powerful and responds by over-reacting—Steven by stepping up his angry pursuit, Matt by exaggerating his demands for distance. By focusing on this endless chase, I highlight what has been hidden by the constant fighting: father and son are deeply involved and deeply affected by each other. They are bound by love and need, masked as mutual recrimination.

In the next segment I use a metaphor, the line that binds fish and fisherman, to clarify the complementarity of their transactions. Humor defuses the emotions, and a good amount of gentle coaching begins to move father and son out of the circle of contact-fight-flight.

M: Steven, do you fish?

STEVEN: No.

M: Because I would say that what Matt does is to bait you. And I wonder why you bite. I don't think that you willfully bait him, Matt, but you do it anyway.

MATT: Why would I try to?

M: I don't know, Matt, I really don't. A person's soul is so obscure that I don't know what the reason is. I just know that you do it, and your father gets hooked every time. Then you get caught in his anger, and you begin to talk obscurely. So how can you get out of that?

MATT: So you're saying I start an argument, huh? I know that's not true. You say I bait him? It's not true.

M: I saw you do it here. I'm certain your father does it, too. You are caught like a fisherman and a fish.

MATT: Well, he baits too!

M: I don't think you feel happy when you're the fish, and I don't think you're happy when you're the fisherman.

MATT: It's different, though, because I don't yell back.

M: No, when you're hooked you talk obscurely. When he feels like a fish, he yells and attacks, and he feels all tied up in knots inside. The question is, will somebody cut the line? Somebody has to do it. It's a painful experience for both of you.

STEVEN: It's gotten so that I expect that kind of thing to happen. So I really don't have any patience.

M: But do you understand that Matt is saying sometimes he feels like a fish?

MATT: If he's yelling and I'm talking in circles, how is that the same?

M: Are you two interested in getting out of this tangle? Or do you enjoy it?

STEVEN (*laughing*): *I* want to get out of it.

MATT: What does talking in circles have to do with it? Tell me specifically what it is.

M: The question is, do you want to stay there? Because if you do, I won't distract you from your fun.

MATT: (*laughing, clearly enjoying himself*): That's funny, really. I suppose that's what you can learn: talking in circles is a fish.

What began as just one more round in father and son's grim struggle over psychic space has been transformed into a game. This shift of frame made it possible to detoxify both Matt's circumlocutions and his father's tirades by absorbing them into a single metaphor, "talking like a fish." Changing the name of the game challenged both the boy and his father: "Which one of you will cut the line?" The answer came from both quarters, with laughter. This incident marked the beginning of a dramatic change in Matt's behavior and in the family's functioning. It also marked a phase in therapy when the focus moved toward fitting fragments into a larger pattern.

STEVEN: There have been times when I felt you were too lenient—that you left Jim with too much freedom. And you felt I wasn't allowing enough freedom.

JOAN: You mean as far as his coming and going?

STEVEN: Yes, coming and going, how often he has the car, things like that.

JOAN: Okay.

STEVEN: I thought the cars ought to be relegated to a very special thing and he really didn't need his own car. I mean that sort of framework.

JOAN: Because I said as long as he earned the money I didn't think we could say how he spent his money. I still say that.

STEVEN: Your mother and I disagree on that, Jim, to a degree. Maybe not as much as we used to.

M (to Jim): So you become part of a triangle?

JOAN: I don't think we ever discussed that with Jim, this dialog between the two of us.

It is very difficult for any family subsystem to work by itself. Certainly if parents have conflicting views about a child, it is impossible for the child not to feel the pull between them. Joan's ignorance about the workings of her own family is not uncommon.

M: I think also that, inside of you, things work mysteriously, Jim. When Steven gets annoyed at you, do you sometimes think, "Well, Mom would be different," or "My own father is different." Do you seek some help from your mother?

JIM: I don't think of asking for help, or that somebody else would be different toward the matter.

STEVEN: But what you do, Jim, is resolve or decide how you feel by going to your mother. That happens a lot. I'll raise an issue with you or ask you to do something and I won't hear any more about it. Then a couple of days later, I'll bring it up to Joan and find out that you and she talked about it and decided what to do. I'm not saying that what you decided to do makes me unhappy. I'm just saying that there have been lots of times when things sort of got settled by you talking to Joan. I guess that's one of the things I would like to change.

M: So the triangle is also maintained by Jim?

STEVEN: I think so, yes.

Frustrated in his attempts to touch bases with Matt, Steven was also experiencing the rejection of his stepson. I encouraged Steven to talk with Jim.

STEVEN: Maybe I set up some of the limits myself, but since there's such a tendency for you to talk to your mother rather than me and since you obviously prefer to talk to Joan rather than me, I'm not as direct with you as I'd like to be. I would like you to be my friend. What I'm trying to struggle with here is that I'd like you to be my friend. (*Jim does not respond.*) Do you know what I just said?

JIM: Uh-huh. Basically.

M: Do you know what he's asking you to do? He was talking straight to you and he was asking you something. Are you going to answer?

JIM: I know what he's asking. When he asks me something or I'm stuck, then I should talk to him about it and not Mom.

M: Can you answer him?

JIM: I know what he was saying.

M: So why don't you answer him?

JIM: The way I got it, I didn't get a question out of it. He just said the way he felt.

It is clear now how Jim and Steven got locked into this particular step. Joan's presence as the third corner of an unacknowledged triangle retarded the development of their relationship. As long as she was available as a comfortable go-between, no new ground would be broken. As a consequence, the two were as uneasy and unfamiliar with each other as they were when they began living together three years ago.

The development of new relationships in blended families may be handicapped by unequal degrees of closeness of its members. Jim and Joan had fifteen years of history before Steven's entry into their lives, as well as hundreds of years of norms defining their mother-son relation. Jim and Steven have nothing on which to draw but a few years of sharing a household; so they must self-consciously define the terms of their relationship if anything real is to develop between them. This requires a kind of delicate collaboration that is easily disrupted by the old affiliations. Steven was not free to reach out to Jim in his own style.

I blocked Joan's subtle involvement many times during this session, to facilitate direct involvement between father and stepson. As they both began to experience the rewards of this new dialog, it became possible to assign them a task. Jim was in the long, painful process of exploring colleges and planning his applications. He was putting off, out of ignorance and anxiety, a problem that was of great concern to Steven and Joan. I asked Steven to work with Jim on college applications, and Joan to validate the task by not responding to Jim in this area. By the last session Jim had three applications almost ready to mail, and the two men were exploring their mutual interest in cars with a warmth that seemed to please them both.

The next exchanges come from the sixth session. Notice that Matt's participation is very different from the first session. He asks permission to enter a dialog between Joan and Steven, and his communication is more direct and appropriate. We were discussing the definition of who parents whom.

M (to Joan): Steven hears that you have a rule. It says, "My son is my particular territory."

JOAN: We talked about it before. I don't think . . .

M: These rules are stated in such small ways that you really don't know how they come to be. Did you hear something from Steven about how to deal with his children?

JOAN: Well, yes, I did. I don't now.

M: What was it?

JOAN: Well, it wasn't a verbal thing. It was again something I felt, something I sensed from his actions, and it was that I was overreaching, overcorrecting Matt. I got the impression that I really shouldn't correct him at all. We worked it out. But I know that in the beginning I refused to talk about it.

STEVEN: Could you be a little more specific?

JOAN: When I would correct Matt, you didn't like it. You'd make excuses for him instead.

STEVEN: I just thought you were too short.

MATT: What does that mean? Or is this a dialog?

M: No, no, you're part of it.

STEVEN: I used to think that Joan was too short, too quick to correct, too sarcastic.

JOAN: I don't think I was sarcastic with Matt.

MATT: I feel you were. Times when you were angry I remember you were . . .

M: Do you see the same thing going on with you, Jim? Your mother felt that Steven was too short with you and sent messages that he shouldn't be. Steven felt that she didn't understand Matt, his child. This is a parallel kind of process.

MATT (*to Steven*): That's over with now, but in the beginning, Dad, I got the impression that you thought I should adjust, change over to Joan's rules. Bedtime, for instance. I changed. I found life was different, somewhat traumatic.

STEVEN: What was traumatic, Matt?

MATT: The fact that the bedtime was changed. I was adjusting, but I thought we were adopting Joan's ways. I didn't feel as though we were combining the two. I thought that you and I were changing into hers.

STEVEN: I know. We talked. I can remember talking to you about it and asking you to try to cooperate and be reasonable. I remember that.

M: This is interesting, Steven. Matt felt that both you and he needed to accommodate more.

MATT: I did. But I felt extreme loyalty to my own family. I still feel it was really rather short timing. It's sort of split us apart, now that I think about it.

M: You said you had a loyalty to the other family. Is this your family now?

MATT: Um, concretely yes. You know, it's set up as that, but I still feel the loyalty for the other one.

STEVEN: You use the word loyalty, Matt—what do you mean by that?

MATT: I can't just erase the old family.

M: Do you feel sometimes that you're betrayed by your father? Do you feel he doesn't support you when you're in disagreement with Joan?

MATT: I guess I tend to when I'm angry, yes.

M: Should he be on your side?

MATT: Well, I'm thinking that if you had been on my side all the time at the beginning, we would have grown further and further apart. We wouldn't all have fit in, if you had been on my side. But when I'm angry, I feel I'm being jumped on.

JOAN: Ganged up on?

MATT: Right.

M: It's the same thing Jim said before. Both of you are operating in terms of the new marriage as a betrayal.

MATT: I guess if you want to say that, yeah. I don't think so now, since I'm somewhere in the middle between anger and content.

As is natural, both parents initially tried to control the new spouse's access to their own child. After all, previous common history makes parent and child adept in reading each other. The new spouse is analphabetic in their language. Slowly, access to the newcomers must build. In the Smith family, this process was different for the two half-families. While Steven and Jim could not develop an autonomous relationship, Joan and Matt drew close together and then blew apart. Many elements may have contributed to these scenarios. Differences in the nature of the original dyads may have led to different outcomes when a third party entered. Similarly, differences between Joan and Steven in their approach to a new stepson created different kinds of resistance—while Joan actively pursued Matt, Steven passively observed Jim. Most important, perhaps, was the difference in the developmental level of the two boys. Jim was an older adolescent, actively consolidating his sense of identity within a social network of peers; Matt, two years younger, was still engaged in an intense struggle to untangle himself from his father so that he could expand. So it is not surprising that Jim's response to the dislocating experience of shifting family allegiances and households was to accelerate his distancing maneuvers, while Matt responded by amplifying the intensity of his stormy struggles with both parents.

The family members' contradictory agendas, which necessarily create conflict and anxiety for all families, are intensified by the circumstances of blended families. For the Smith family, autonomy versus belonging was recast as a struggle between the new parents and the children, a struggle not only over proximity and distance but over past and present. The parents said, in effect, "Join up." (Steven recollects that he told Matt to "cooperate and be reasonable," and Joan recalls that she told Matt she wanted to "make up for what his real mother didn't give him.")

For children, such a message can be experienced as a negation, not only of their past memories and experiences but of their current reality. Children in blended families are often operating in a much more complex field than their parents. They may be active participants of two family systems, sometimes shuttling between two households, or at least maintaining contact with the remnants of the old family system and whatever additional membership that group has developed. If the new spouses push the children to accommodate to the new family, rather than permit them to evolve a complex solution to a complex problem, the children may well respond by "freezing in place." Put another way, to the extent that the parents are asking them to negate the past, they will refuse to accept the present. In the Smith family both boys saw their parents' marriage as a betrayal. Clearly they both experienced the pressure to accommodate to the new family not as a four-way collaboration, but as a negation of their own family's subculture, as a triumph for the culture of the "other side."

At the end of the seventh session, I suggested that the parents share some of their life experiences as adolescents with both children. This is something parents enjoy doing with their own children, and in blended families it can be a way of constructing necessary pathways, since the family must build a common history in a telescoped time. Joan and Steven reported the results in the eighth session, the last one. The grim tension of the early sessions had given way to a lighter mood.

STEVEN: We talked about the experiences I had in school. Real quickly, what it amounted to was I had skipped a year in grade school. So I felt kind of out of place, because I was a year younger than the other kids. I wanted to make friends so my way of making friends was to find the fellows in the class that got the most attention. I wanted to be one of them. If someone threw an eraser—that's how I developed my joining into the group. We talked about that, and Joan talked about some of her experiences.

M: You were telling Matt that long long ago you were young people also.

JOAN: Steven and I were talking, and Matt became interested.

M: Were they interesting, Matt?

MATT: I thought so. They're human.

M: You didn't know that?

MATT: You can't help that they were young only before you were born, right?

M: Yes, that's usually how it works.

MATT: You realize they're more human when you know they weren't good little kids.

M: Is that helpful?

MATT: Yeah. I can feel more at home and talk easier. Last night . . .

STEVEN: I wasn't upset with you last night.

MATT: I know, but you were yelling at me, you know, "Put the jumper cables down."

STEVEN: I was angry at Jim and Jim wasn't there to get it, and you were. So I wasn't yelling at you, the tone of my voice was . . .

MATT: I didn't feel like I had before. I realized it was Jim's fault. I just stood there and I was quiet.

STEVEN: Yes, I appreciated that, as I thought about it afterwards. If you had complained it would have started contributing to the problem. Yet you left me alone, let me rant for a little while, and then it went away.

MATT: I tried to be helpful.

M: You don't need me! You're at the point where you can heal your father. You don't need me.

People do not learn a new language in eight hours. Nonetheless, the Smiths were speaking in a different tongue. My goal as a coach of families in transition—not to teach something new but to give a different perspective on their reality—was achieved. Patterns shifted, and old skills could suddenly be put to use in an expanded way.

READER: I think I understand why you chose these families in transition. But, you know, I'm still concerned about the traditional family. What will become of . . .

AUTHOR: The traditional family will remain what it is now—one of many possible family shapes. And I don't know that what we're seeing is all that new. I live in a traditional family: my wife and I have two children, the older a son, and we've been married for thirty-two years. But in fact—we say it in jest, but it's quite true—we've been divorced and remarried thirty times, maybe more. Each time a new possibility.

READER: That's interesting. As I read "Trio," I was sure you had divorced and remarried. You seemed determined to gloss over the difficulties and focus on the possibilities.

AUTHOR: You're right. But the reason is that families are organisms in a continuous process of changing while trying to remain the same. You can mourn the structure that was lost, but it makes more sense to look at the possibilities of the new. I recently lost my mother. I am sixty-two, and she was eighty-two. Since then I've put her picture of my grandparents on my desk, and realize with pain that the tradition my mother remembered has died with her. My memories have shrunk, I have become less. But, with my mother's death, my wife and I have become the oldest generation, and I suddenly experience with pleasure my children's protection. With time we will heal and there will be new connections, especially with my brother and sister. We will become grandparents, and with time and change will come crisis, transition, possibilities.

READER: I'm sorry about your mother. I understand what you're getting at. You believe in growth through experimentation. You're pushing hope.

AUTHOR: Better than pushing drugs.

READER: Are you a hope addict?

AUTHOR: I do believe we are all underfunctioning, tremendously.

READER: Let me understand. You think a systemic perspective may correct that? That the acceptance of being a part of a larger whole may challenge individual rigidities and, paradoxically, induce individual growth? That an understanding of complementarity might bring harmony?

AUTHOR: And humility, less wear and tear, less blame and aggression—yes.

READER: Now you sound more like a preacher than a social scientist.

AUTHOR: I have rabbis in my ancestry. But I'm not talking about the righteous life, only about epistemological change. You know, it is possible to recognize oneself as belonging. I've always felt part of patterns—a part of my home town in Argentina, imbedded in its rural geography, a member of the Jewish Minuchin clan, son and brother, bound to and competitor of my childhood friends, nephew, cousin, husband, father. I've always felt connected. Haven't you?

READER: Of course in this framing all I can do is respond with my own connectives—the important people in my past who still persist in me. But we differ, because I experience them as constraints, as responsibility, even control.

AUTHOR: That's a trick of punctuation. We are always constructing our present and reconstructing our past, erasing commas, adding new exclamation points. Our culture promotes selfhood, so we tend to blur our connections.

READER: You have an easy time with reality. You seem to arrange facts to support your statements, as if everything were perspective.

AUTHOR: Perspective is reality from a certain position, and vice versa. You see, something happened to my thinking when I began to see people in context. I learned to question the boundaries of myself, and even to feel a certain kinship with wasps and bees.

READER: But you're the most important.

AUTHOR: Yes, of course. I know it's not true, but I can't help feeling that way.

READER: Everybody does. Can you really see yourself as a part? A fragment?

AUTHOR: You've trapped me. I do feel I am the center of the universe, an island unto myself. But I know this is craziness and that in reality I'm only a fragment in a kaleidoscope. One tiny turn, and I become a spot in another pattern.

READER: Well, I guess I know that too, though it's not precisely a comfortable thought. Let's return to the blended family. Is it one of the turnings in the kaleidoscope of today's culture?

AUTHOR: I think so. It seems to be performing some of the functions of the extended family. The difference is that in our culture the framework is horizontal. Let me show you two scenes from my own family today.

Amy, the daughter of our niece Ellen, is very excited, preparing for her father's third marriage. She and her paternal half-sister will be the flower girls at the wedding. Amy also has a stepsister Jill, daughter of her stepfather, with whom she plays every other weekend when Jill comes to visit her father. So Amy, though an only child, feels very close to her two "siblings," and she wonders if her father will have a son, since she is both uneasy and pleased at the idea of having a brother.

Recently I went to the funeral of my wife's cousin, a man I admired. His third wife and their children were seated in the first row of chairs; his first wife and one of their daughters were in the last; his second wife did not come, but near the middle row sat a woman friend with whom he had lived for most of his last years. These three "families" shared memories and mourning. Given needs, society finds a solution.

READER: It's a solution that doesn't work very smoothly yet.
AUTHOR: That's because we have no rituals. We have no traditions or guidelines for families to blend in mourning, for instance, as participants in some kind of collective *shiva*. The support systems these horizontal families can provide are still a product of pure improvisation and good will. Perhaps in the not too distant future we will develop "blending ceremonies" to encourage the maintenance of supportive relationships among segments of families who have shared members. It would be worth a try.

The Key

Fragmentation of a Commune

The 1960s produced a strange crusade. A world army was formed, called to arms by word of mouth, and from the remote corners of the planet, from attics and cellars, dark bars and sunny beaches, soldiers armed with a flower and a smile marched on an unsuspecting world under the banner of goodness. LSD and pot were part of the crusade, but not of the essence; they were merely the artifacts that would allow the world to recognize the truth of the dream. Colors would become truer, we would return to the unblemished capacity to touch and feel. Time would pulsate and curve as Einstein said it does, and people would discover people.

In Paris a collection of old names dreamed of joining flowered youth by becoming the strategists of the movement. R. D. Laing proposed putting LSD in Manhattan's water reservoir to observe the dreams in Wall Street the next day. (Perhaps he did.) In the Dam Platze in Amsterdam hundreds of youths from all over the world were provided by the city with information on centers where help was given if they had a bad trip. New messiahs like Timothy Leary prayed to the sign of the mushroom, and throngs of youth dreamed wings and flew toward the sun; for others, the dreams became nightmares.

In the late sixties I was in Amsterdam to give a seminar in family therapy. The student therapists, some fifteen of them, brought families in treatment for consultation. I joined the therapists in sessions and, in a mixture of English and translated Dutch, tried to be helpful to the family and students in the expanded time of the therapeutic session. Joss was a therapist of the times. He had long hair, wore jeans before jeans were designed by Cardin, and a shirt with a polo neck. He took off his shoes and entered a room like a black-belt master. He sat in the lotus position and moved sometimes by balancing his body on his hands, sometimes by jumping to his feet and moving around the room until he found the right spot to center himself again in the lotus position. He watched me for five days and decided that I could be trusted, despite my age. He was going to bring in for consultation a Marxist commune: four people who called themselves a family and wanted to be seen as a unit.

The problem presented by the group was Mary's migraines. They had started a few months ago and made her life miserable. In a strange way, these migraines had become a political problem; Mary requested a room of her own, or at least privacy during her attacks. This meant a key to the door, hence private space, hence capitalism. The young people were bright, beautiful, full of dreams. They were championing a new concept in family organization and were suspicious of my age, my profession, and my reputation. I wanted to be accepted, or at least to impress them. I took a volume of *Das Kapital* from the distant shelves of my memory and began to parry with Tom and Jim. They were better than I was, but they accepted my effort. Maybe they could postpone their mistrust until I finished showing my wares.

The quartet's problem was evident to me after ten minutes: there were two males, attracted to the lovely Mary, and a second female trying not to notice. Mary was at the center of a suppressed emotional storm. Her solution was to develop migraines, a neat way to achieve distance without challenging the balance of the commune. The response of the men was chauvinistic (had this term been coined yet?), not to mention psychologically naive. They insisted that Mary had to overcome her feminine vapors.

I remember asking Mary to sit in a low chair and then moving the chair from one place to another (I was stronger then), treating her as an object. I developed this theme and challenged the group, in the name of Marx, to accept the individual needs of their members.

Now I draw a blank; I don't remember what happened next. Perhaps the clock struck midnight, and I suddenly changed back into a middle-aged psychiatrist, married to the same woman for fifteen years. Perhaps my psychological challenge was accordingly dismissed as capitalistic propaganda. I simply don't know. That's one of the frustrations of being a consultant. You start a process, but you don't know how it evolves. I always have the feeling that I left the theater after the first act.

Of course, I don't want pat endings. Even as a child, I hated the movie cowboy's habit of riding off into the sunset, leaving the girl he had just kissed alone and defenseless on the open prairie. One of my favorite games then was to invent more story, and years later I still indulge in the same pastime. It is in that vein that question marks about the commune arise. Is it still, seventeen years later, a viable organism, its members older and perhaps wiser? Or did they (like so many of the communes of the sixties) move with the times to find some other family organization? What follows is one of the possibilities. "The Key" is dedicated to the flower children, the heroes of surely the strangest crusade in recent history. With my thanks and respect.

The Key

Scene 1

(*The set has three rooms. The center room is a kitchen-dining-living room and the side rooms are two smaller bedrooms, each one with a double bed, a chair, and a closet. In the room at the left Mary is lying in bed in semi-darkness. The one on the right is lighted, and Jane is lying in bed reading. The apartment is neat and clean with posters of Picasso's* Guernica *and the dove of peace; good furniture mingles with thrift-shop specials.*

When the play starts, Tom and Jim are in the center room. Tom is preparing a salad, cutting up vegetables. He is very slow and methodical. Jim is setting the table. The men are careful in their preparations, as if it were a special occasion.)

TOM (*in mid-lecture*): We *are* prisoners, with only the illusion of freedom. We fill our life with things.

JIM (*indicating items on the table as he talks*): Lighted candles, wine and glasses, white tablecloth, our best china.

TOM: Seriously, Jim (*begins to cut onions precisely*), we were hypnotized as children. (*The onions make his eyes water, and he cleans his glasses with a napkin.*) We still carry our parents' concepts of reality.

JIM (*kidding*): You shouldn't become so emotional when you talk about your parents. You'll cry in the salad.

TOM (*wiping his eyes and smiling*): Okay, funny guy, if you've finished setting the table, go and see if Mary's headache has improved. Dinner will be ready soon.

(*Jim goes to the room on the left, walking on tiptoe, opens the door gently, puts his head in and sees Mary sitting up. He enters the room and sits silently on the chair for thirty seconds.*)

JIM (*softly*): How are you feeling?

MARY: Much better. It's just a migraine. If I stay alone for half an hour with my eyes closed, it goes away. (*Jim massages her temples, then her forehead; Mary smiles. As she speaks she is vivacious, full of energy.*) You know, it's almost a forced Zen experience. (*Lightly*) "Concentrate on a point in front of you." Sometimes people look funny, like Giacometti's people—the faces and bodies narrow, the movements delayed, like in a world of puppets. It used to scare me, but now—

JIM: Do you think that joining the commune has been too rough on you? I feel guilty because I pushed you into it.

MARY: No, Jim, you didn't push me. I joined *with* you. I like challenging the world of flat people.

JIM: Well, it was okay a year ago when we joined. But now I have the feeling that I pushed you into doing something you didn't want. The truth is that belonging is easier in the abstract. (*He massages her shoulders and forehead; she smiles and relaxes.*)

(*In the central room, Tom continues cooking; after finishing the salad, he breaks eight eggs in a bowl and beats them. Jane stops reading, closes the book, and goes to the center room.*)

TOM (*indicating the other room with his head*): Jim is helping Mary with her headache. I think she may shoot holes in our life.

JANE: Do you think her headaches are psychological?

TOM: No, just petit-bourgeois. But this business of having a key to one room will destroy this family! We're a social animal, not an aggregate of people (*he beats the eggs with savage energy*).

JANE (*as if reciting a well-learned lesson*): We are one. I am a part of you. But your experiment needs people who share your vision.

TOM (*patronizing*): Jane, it's not "my experiment." I didn't get enlightenment by watching a proletarian bee screwing the queen bee and then dying. It's quite simple. If we abolish ownership, if we don't own, we belong. We share and are shared.

JANE: You can't expect Mary to understand you . . .

TOM (*abruptly*): I think dinner will be ready soon. (*He concentrates on the cooking, and Jane goes to get her book, and comes back to read on the couch. In the other room, Mary opens her eyes and smiles.*)

MARY: I feel okay now, thanks. I think we were right in joining. The world would be better if people didn't transform each other into dollar signs. (*Looks at Jim.*) How much are you worth, Jim, in the open market?

JIM: You're a good pupil of Professor Tom.

MARY: I think he's right. I just think he's wrong in making all this fuss about the key for the bedroom. I only need it to close myself in when I have a headache. How will my staying alone a couple of hours affect the future of humanity?

JIM: You know what Tom says—if we divide the space, we let our parents in.

MARY: Fuck Professor Tom, always so absolutely right (*begins to tease Jim in bed*). Do you think it will be selfish of us if we have our orgasms out of sync with them?

JIM: We won't tell them the precise time.

MARY (*pouncing on him*): That is rebellion, my dear Jim! You've become an ally of American capitalism.

JIM (*pushing her back*): Not now. They're waiting for us to start the meeting. (*Mary tickles him and they wrestle.*)

TOM (*pouring milk into the eggs*): If she owns a key, she owns a door. She separates. She manipulates our space and we get swallowed by her boundaries.

JANE (*looking at the book*): How can she do that, Tom? The group is larger than its parts.

TOM: It's the idea of one of us trying to control us all. If we accept a traffic cop, it's the end of the experiment. (*Mary and Jim come in.*)

JIM: It's not the end—it's the first anniversary of the family (*goes to the table and lights a candle*). Happy birthday to all of us!

(*Tom takes off the cooking apron, cleans his hands, and comes to the center of the room. Jane closes her book and joins. The four embrace around the waist and form a circle; they begin slowly to turn. They turn three times in one direction and three times opposite.*)

ALL (*chanting*): The circle is the center of life; the circle is the beginning and the end; there is no guilt and no shame since we are one. (*They stop and arrange four cushions on the floor. They sit with their arms touching, forming a square.*)

TOM (*intoning*): The square is the perfect geometric figure. Four is a perfect human structure. Today, the sixth of May, 1968, in the age of our parents, but day one of the year two of our commune, as secretary I open our meeting. Who wants to talk?

MARY (*defiantly*): We have from the last meeting the unresolved issue of a key for one room.

TOM: You still on that?

MARY: Yes, I am.

TOM: You are threatening the fabric of our society.

MARY: I don't want to do that, but my headaches improve if I lie in the dark for half an hour or so. I don't know how you can equate that with capitalism.

TOM: When you demand space, you introduce the delusion that each one of us is a whole . . .

MARY (*firmly*): I don't want to reject anybody. I just want to be alone when I have headaches.

TOM: Is it possible that your parents' house, with the room for the maid, and the six bathrooms, is still your model of the real world? (*Tom and Mary begin to glare at each other like two boxers ready to pounce.*)

JIM (*sarcastic*): Does it occur to you that you sound like a preacher? What's Mary's crime? She has headaches. What does she ask? Some space of her own. How will this destroy our combined enlightenment?

TOM: Jim (*getting up*), a key to a door puts a label on a room. You and Mary get one bedroom, and Jane and I the other, and we get separated into two couples. And when I have sex with Mary in your bedroom we cuckold you.

JIM (*stands up and faces Tom*): As always, Professor, your logic is perfect. It's your humanity that's lacking. I go to the girls *only* if they want me. If Mary or Jane wants to be alone, I'm alone too.

JANE (*looking up*): But the truth, Jim, is that you visit Mary more than me. Don't you like me?

MARY: Jane, what kind of shit is this? Are you the female possession of the two commissars?

TOM: That's unfair. I respect Jane.

MARY (*standing up*): You're a capitalist! You have two cows and milk them to exhaustion and when one is tired, you demand (*yelling*) the right of the owner! We are objects you move (*takes a cushion and throws it. She pulls Tom to the couch and straddles him*). Do you want me like this or (*turns around and sits on him*) or like this (*lies down on the floor opening her legs*), like this, or (*crouching, her behind high*) like this?

JIM (*protective and soothing*): God, calm yourself, Mary. You've made your point. Tom is wrong.

MARY: It's not just Tom. It's also you, Jim. Jane and I aren't full partners in this experiment of yours. We're just . . . the women. So tell me, why do I have to share only you and Tom? What about Jane? (*Puts her arms around Jane.*) You see yourself as less attractive than me only because Tom hovers around me. But if this is really a commune, who decided it has to be heterosexual?

JANE (*alarmed*): I don't understand you.

TOM (*pedantically*): Look, Mary, our shape is a geodesic structure. You put slack in one corner or too much pull in another, and the whole deck of cards will tumble down.

MARY: That's why you're afraid of change, Professor.

TOM: Yes, we can only control the beginning of change.

MARY (*looking at Jim*): But we joined the family because it offered new possibilities for change.

TOM: Only within its rules.

JANE (*sitting on the couch near Tom*): I don't think I've changed. I embraced Tom and moved in sync with him. I don't see changes, because our distances remain the same.

MARY (*sitting on the floor on a cushion, next to Jim*): Are you saying that you joined just to be close to Tom?

JANE: Yes. I'm no intellectual. I love Tom, so I know he's right. When I was young I was afraid of the dark. To go to sleep I would concentrate on a wrinkle in the pillowcase. Then you could take me in my bed anyplace in the world. As long as the point in my pillowcase went with me, *I* didn't move.

MARY: Are you putting me on?

JANE: No! Listen, many people travel through the world—India, Australia, Africa—always staying in the same Holiday Inn.

TOM: Actually, I focus only on the essentials too. Then you're at the center, the world moves and you don't.

JIM: But you run the risk of restricting yourself.

TOM: Not in *my* book. It depends on what you see as essentials. I choose two major truths, Marxism and Zen. With them, a toothbrush, a set of underwear, I'm at home wherever I am.

MARY: You confuse me. Are you saying the world doesn't exist?

TOM: Of course. *You* are my world. This is why I'm afraid of any changes. Our family is frail; any tampering with it, and we're in free-fall.

MARY (*to Jim*): Am I wrong, or is Tom double-talking? Is he a conservative masquerading as a Zen-Marxist?

TOM: Of course I'm a conservative. We made the revolution when we rejected our parents' world. Now it's essential to maintain it, and *your key* is threatening our world.

JIM: *I* think a few changes, like a key in Mary's door, can't threaten our growth.

TOM: You're naive. We're still a new animal, a mutant, and the world outside is hostile.

MARY: What do we do, then? Stick ourselves at this junction, a Cezanne still life preserving its flat peaches forever?

TOM: What would you suggest?

MARY (*stands up*): I don't know yet, but I know this: if I need time out, I should have it, and we'll take a new form for a while. I know it will please Jane—she's been jealous of the three of us.

JANE: Being at a certain distance while you three were close is a kind of variation I accepted.

MARY: But do you like it?

JANE: I accept it.

MARY: Jane, goddamit, do you like it?

JANE: I know it will change at its correct time.

MARY: Well, hallelujah! The correct time is *now*. I need distance *now*.

TOM: Mary, you want to impose your will on the group.

MARY: I don't want *you* to impose yours.

TOM: Why do you say that?

MARY: Because you want me and Jim to be at your side with Jane distant. (*She positions Tom, Jim, and Jane, with Jane separate.*)

TOM: Not really. I'd like to be surrounded by all of you. (*He brings Jane in front of him.*)

MARY: *You* at the center of everybody!

TOM: No, *me,* being protected by all of you.

JIM (*to Mary*): What arrangement would you prefer?

TOM: Is this a vote?

JIM: Something like that. Mary? (*Mary arranges Jim three feet from her, Tom five feet, then goes to Jane and brings her two feet from her.*)

TOM: I don't believe you.

MARY: You prefer your own version.

JIM: You can't accept that Mary is closer to me.

MARY: But I also want the alternative (*moves back several feet*), to step back when I have my migraines.

JIM: Jane, what kind of arrangement do you want?

JANE (*recreates Tom's arrangement*): This one.

MARY: With Tom or you at the center?

JANE: It really doesn't matter.

MARY: It matters to me, Jane. Don't you see what's happened? You've lost yourself.

JANE: I know where I am.

MARY: You don't know who you are. Don't you see, this commune is controlled by them. We've lived for so long in man-country that we've accepted their rules. (*Brings Jane to the couch, sits close, touching her.*) Jane, you have a capacity to give, and to belong, that neither Tom nor Jim has. Tom calls it "femininity," and you bought that (*caresses her hair, her face*), and so did I. We accepted the niches they constructed for us. But I see you in a different light. The more you give, the more you seem to grow.

JANE (*crying and holding Mary's hands while Mary strokes her hair*): Mary, this is beautiful. (*Slowly Mary pulls Jane to her feet and they go to one of the bedrooms; Mary opens the door, turns toward Tom and Jim.*)

MARY: We don't want dinner. Good night.

JANE (*turning around, smiling*): Good night. (*Closes the door.*)

TOM: Well, it seems Mary found her key.

(*As the women enter the right-hand bedroom, they put on the light and sit on the bed. They hold hands, look at each other hesitantly. They talk quietly. In the center room, Tom and Jim look at each other, surprised by the speed of the events.*)

JIM: Happy birthday, Tom.

TOM: It doesn't make any sense.

JIM: But it happened . . . in front of our eyes. Mary seduced Jane.

TOM: Jane is a follower. She clings to a stronger person, and if the other moves, she thinks she has too.

JIM: Yes, Jane is easy to understand, but I don't get Mary. We both know she enjoys sex. (*Enumerating with his fingers*) She fools around screwing, she likes to explore new positions, she has strong vaginal orgasms.

TOM: Well, she's not like that with me . . . actually she's rather passive. I am always on top of her and she doesn't come every time. But I agree with you—she's very feminine, and for her to go after Jane seems an act of spite.

JIM: Goddamit, what a waste!

(*In the other room, the lights go out.*)

TOM: Look what they've done to us.

JIM: I see what they've done—(*angry*) left us out in the cold, with both of them closeted, drinking the ambrosia of their own tits.

TOM: Don't you see the challenge? Mary has thrown us a curve ball. What do we do with it?

JIM: What do you mean?

TOM: Mary has thrown down her gauntlet. She and Jane are exploring homosexuality. (*A change in his voice*) Mary is saying *we* are self-sufficient. (*Very slowly*) You . . . have . . . each . . . other.

JIM: Yes (*thoughtfully*), for sure.

TOM (*looking tense, rubbing his hands together slowly*): Intellectually, she's right. If we are a revolutionary figure, the distant angles should find a way of touching.

JIM (*perceiving the change in Tom*): Professor, are you saying we should screw each other? (*Short laugh.*)

TOM: No, not screwing . . . (*softly*) though it was part of the Greek patrician life.

JIM (*getting up*): Well, I am not Greek (*continues with a forced lightness that contrasts with the quiet seriousness of Tom*). Besides I go for the six-foot blond primitive type. But, really, why are you taking Mary so seriously?

TOM: Because you're getting more and more anxious. Sit down.

JIM (*sarcastically*): Now comes the psychoanalysis bit! You're stretching it too far. I'd better go to sleep. (*He goes into the left room, closes the door, takes a chair, buttresses the door.*)

(*Tom gets up, turns off the light, and throws himself on the couch.*)

TOM (*in the dark*): He didn't understand.

Scene 2

(*Next day. Tom is sleeping on the couch, covered by a blanket. Mary and Jane enter the middle room. Jane looks more assertive, her hair is done differently. They begin to make breakfast. Tom opens his eyes.*)

JANE: Did you sleep well?

TOM: Not a wink the whole night, just tossed and turned, waiting for breakfast.

(*Mary goes to Jim's door, tries to open it but can't. She looks at Tom.*)

MARY: Does Jim have a lock?

(*Jim, in the other room, pulls the chair away from the door and opens it.*)

JIM: Hi! (*Smiles, uncomfortably.*)

MARY (*friendly*): We're making breakfast. Wash and come in.

JIM: Okay. (*Goes into the bathroom.*)

(*Tom has turned his back as the women prepare breakfast. Jim goes back to his room; Tom goes into the bathroom. They both come and sit at the table, without looking at each other.*)

MARY (*to Jane*): You go and sit with them. I'll finish here. Tom, Jim, scrambled eggs?

TOM (*smiling*): You can use the eggs we didn't use last night.

MARY: No, today is the beginning of a new era.

JANE (*sitting with Tom and Jim*): I'm sorry if we dealt you a crooked hand of cards last night.

JIM: You can say that again.

TOM: What happens now?

JANE: I'm afraid I have a surprise for you.

JIM: I know. You and Mary are pregnant (*laughs*).

MARY (*from the kitchen, smiling*): Not a bad double play.

TOM (*concerned*): What's the surprise, Jane?

JANE: I'm leaving the group today. (*Mary brings mugs of coffee.*)

TOM (*speaks hurriedly, swallowing endings*): I half expected it, but why? Why today? Why don't you stay, Jane? What happened last night?

JANE: Nothing happened last night, except I found out who I am.

TOM: Are you saying you found out you're lesbian?

JANE: Not actually. The sex part wasn't that good. She stinks as a lover. No, I found out I'm a person.

TOM: That's quite an indictment of me.

JANE: No, Tom, we collaborated. As I clung to you, you made all the decisions. In the end, I became your shadow.

JIM: What was last night—magic?

JANE: Mary . . . she really is an amazing person, Jim. She made me feel wanted. She . . . laughed at my jokes. My God, nobody's laughed at my jokes since I was eight years old. We didn't sleep all night. At three in the morning, I was telling stories about my adolescence . . . my dreams . . . and I began to listen to myself. I was an interesting, involved, curious person. What did I do to myself? And Mary was there—she just listened and I felt confirmed. It was the most wonderful night of my life. Just all at once I stretched out.

TOM: What do you plan to do when you leave?

JANE: I was afraid you'd be angry.

TOM: Of course, I'm angry, and hurt. Mary and her goddammed key! Like the trumpets of Joshua, it's destroying our world.

JANE: It wasn't Mary, Tom. We've all changed.

(*Mary comes with eggs and serves around the table.*)

JIM (*gets up, in a mocking tone*): The magician. So (*to Jane*), where are you going?

JANE: To my parents' house for a while. It's funny how we always think of them as available when we're down and narrow-minded when we're up. I think I'll go pack. (*To Tom*) I've got to leave now, before you convince me not to. (*She goes to the room on the right and starts her packing.*)

(*The three others look at each other, in silence. They smile, playing with objects on the table.*)

JIM: Well, that's that.

TOM: What do we do now?

MARY: I wonder if a trio can function.

TOM: No (*looking where Jane had been sitting*), a triangle is only half a square. I don't think it can work.

MARY: What are *you* going to do?

TOM (*stands*): I just made a decision. I'll leave today as well—I don't know where I'll go, (*lightly*) but I own a toothbrush and some underwear.

MARY (*looking at Jim*): Well, that leaves *us* together. Just like old times.

JIM: Not really, Mary. I got a jolt last night.

MARY: Anything happen between you and Tom?

JIM: No . . . nothing. I just need time alone. (*Mary looks at him alarmed.*) I'll be back . . . one or two weeks at most. (*He gets up and slowly goes to his room.*)

MARY: Two weeks . . . two months . . . two years. (*She picks up Tom's mug and spills coffee on the table in a circle, then takes the other mug and spills coffee on the floor around her chair, like a dog marking territory, leaving herself enclosed. She sits with a forlorn, little-girl expression and drinks her own coffee.*) Shit!

(*Curtain*)

READER: Are you implying that communes are not viable organisms?

AUTHOR: Not at all. Just that I don't think that one was. Its members saw themselves as individuals, but their ideologies blinded them to individual needs, making the organism nonviable.

READER: Why did you select homosexuality as the trigger of crisis in that commune? In the Marxist frame . . .

AUTHOR: For precisely that reason: to highlight the need for congruity between human process and imposed conceptual models. There are limits, you know, to the flexibility of social systems. Ideologists frequently dismiss those limitations as the constructs of weak-minded wishy-washy liberals.

READER: You're getting rhetorical all of a sudden. Why?

AUTHOR: That frequently happens to me when I'm challenging, and become afraid of the consequences of a line of thought. Let me try again. Family members develop, through continuous interaction, a shared frame of reality. This common model filters everyone's experience, and consequently it both restrains and facilitates growth. The process of building that frame is slow, repetitive, selective, confusing, and frequently illogical. But the results are always idiosyncratic, and the vision is always tailor-made to the specifications of that particular group. Ideologies, on the other hand, are explanations of universals. They are logical, all-encompassing, clear, and in theory representative of encompassing truth. Talmudists, Jesuits, the self-styled right-to-lifers, politicians—ideologues of any sort (including psychiatrists, of course)—insist on their own ownership of truth, and on the infinite capacity of human systems to receive and respond to that truth.

READER: Are you really saying that Mary's homosexual experimentation was as much an expression of ideology as Tom's Marxism?

AUTHOR: Of course.

READER: But she must have had some lesbian leanings.

AUTHOR: Maybe, maybe not. It might have been a response to the organization of the commune.

READER: Then why did it precipitate a breakup?

AUTHOR: Well, there's a rather humbling concept in systems

thinking having to do with change. The crux of the idea is that while you can initiate, you can't entirely predict consequences.

READER: Given the interconnectedness of people in a system, change in one person will be reflected in other system members.

AUTHOR: Yes, but more than that—sometimes small inputs produce large results. There's no way of covering all the angles.

READER: What's the use of a theory that cannot predict? When you're dealing at the individual level, you at least have more manageable sets of variables. And another thing. When you replace the focus on the individual with an exploration of the system, aren't you driving toward anonymity? Tinkering with rather well-defined concepts of self only to give us the mindless complexity of the beehive?

AUTHOR: If you want to talk about beehives—

READER: I don't, actually. Animal analogies seem questionable to me, at best. Let's stick to people. Times Square at 5 p.m., say.

AUTHOR: We're not talking about strangers, though, but about organisms with a common history, sharing space, time, and future.

READER: Look, I know my family influences me. But I remember when I was twelve years old—the light and the darkness of that period. And nobody else in the world shares that. What do *you* do with individual memories?

AUTHOR: I carry and cherish them, just as you do. But, you know, I notice that they change with life. I lose some. Others are expanded and embellished. Some grow with time and perspective. Have you noticed the effect your children have on your memories?

READER: Yes. But I'm still me. Oh, I can understand reciprocal influences—

AUTHOR: You still don't understand.

READER: Are you really talking about a multibodied organism?

AUTHOR: Yes.

READER: Then maybe you're talking about science fiction. I read a story once about five people with different specialties, united by telepathic communication. But to see human beings as—

AUTHOR: Theodore Sturgeon's *More Than Human*. I like that title. It's a different way of seeing, and a perspective, by the way, that enhances the view of the individual rather than curtailing it. But you're right. It goes against all traditional learning and against the way everyone is taught to experience.

READER: Then what makes you think people will change?

AUTHOR: Because they have already.

READER: You mean ecology, cybernetics, "spaceship earth," I suppose?

AUTHOR: More or less.

READER: But there's a big difference between a change in technology that allows a few technicians to handle Telstar cybernetically and the perception of our own families as systems.

AUTHOR: We have always been a little slower in incorporating knowledge into our social frames. But, you know, I think we should move on now. We seem to have reached a plateau. And the next chapter presents one of the best demonstrations of systems effects—the treatment of psychosomatic illness by family therapy.

An Anorectic Family

Repatterning through Therapy

Dear Dr. Minuchin:

I have a daughter who is an anorectic. She is 5′3″ and weighs 80 pounds. The condition was diagnosed a year ago, and she has been hospitalized twice when her weight went below the minimum set by the attending physician. She has been in therapy ever since, but stays pretty much the same. It's creating problems for the whole family: she makes lavish desserts that she insists everybody else has to eat, she drinks all the fruit juice in the refrigerator, hides containers of vomit around the house, and in general, lies about anything and everything connected with her consumption of food and drink.

She is obsessed with exercise and what to eat, when to eat, etc. We do not believe we make any excessive demands on her; in fact, rather the opposite. She is an overachiever, third in her class.

I asked the doctor last week if he felt that she has made any improvement, and his comment was definitely yes, but that it may take one to ten years to straighten everything out. I brought up the subject of behavioral therapy, which I know is quick, but he said it would only remove the anorexia, and if you remove one problem another will surface in its place. He prefers to get to the bottom, the origin, no matter how long that takes.

I feel that if you remove the most harmful problems first, although the underlying one will still be there, certain other pieces of the puzzle might fall into place. At this stage of the game I am totally confused. I am appealing to you. We need help desperately, both for my daughter's health and for the sake of our family . . .

This letter is representative of many I have received over the past fifteen years. As my work with anorexia became known, I heard from many anguished parents.

It started almost by accident, with the appearance of a family who wanted to be seen as a family, because their adolescent son was refusing to eat. His refusal was slow, logical, and even laudable. Coming from a high-minded Quaker family who revered life, he first became a vegetarian to avoid killing, then by a logical extension refused to wear leather shoes and belts. Later he began to avoid all food that didn't contain a seed he could salvage and plant. As a result he was dying slowly, committing suicide in the name of protecting life.

I published a paper on the case in 1970, and pretty soon I had a large number of referrals of anorectic patients, mostly girls of course. They presented rather similar characteristics, being hard-working, perfectionist, nice clean adolescent girls, close to their families, dependent on their mothers, depressed, and obsessively concerned with food and the fear of getting fat. Since I included their families in my therapy, I soon began to realize that they too resembled each other.

Eventually this work with anorectic families became part of a study on psychosomatic illness in children and the use of family therapy in such cases. The research has been described elsewhere. Its relevance here is that by now, when I meet a family with an anorectic child, I am entering known territory. I know that these families have one predominant characteristic: they are enmeshed to the point that boundaries between people are far too weak to define and protect. Anorectic families are trapped in the kind of dependency where commitment, loyalty, and the well-being of the group are paramount. This is a fertile environment for somatic response to psychological stress.

Loretta Genotti, sixteen, is the oldest daughter of a working-class Italian-American family. Her parents came to the United States from Sicily shortly after their marriage. Neither of them completed grammar school, but they are both intelligent and competent people. The father is a postal clerk; the mother is a housewife. Their English is sometimes more rapid than fluent.

When Loretta was fourteen she was admitted to a large city hospital complaining of severe pain in her abdomen. She remained in the hospital for two months, sometimes not eating because of the intense pain. After extensive medical workups, organic causes for the pain were ruled out; the diagnosis: "psychological problems." She refused to see a psychiatrist.

For two years Loretta continued to lose weight and was becoming obsessed with this problem. The diagnosis this time was "simple schizophrenia with superficial depressive features." Thorazine was prescribed. Three months later Loretta was again hospitalized, with the diagnosis of anorexia nervosa. On admission she weighed around 80 pounds. She remained in the hospital for six weeks. Her eating improved, and she gained weight. The continuation of therapy on an outpatient basis was recommended, but the family did not follow through.

Four months later Loretta was again admitted to the hospital—to the intensive care unit. There her condition was stabilized, but she remained in the hospital for another two months with little improvement. Her family signed her out against medical advice. She weighed 75 pounds. Eating problems continued. She was amenorrheic and depressed. She had not attended school for some months.

Somehow Mrs. Genotti learned that I was going to present a case consultation at a community mental-health outpatient clinic. Recognizing my name from a recent popular article on anorexia nervosa, she wrote to me, volunteering her family for the consultation. Her learning of the consultation, advertised only among professionals, gives some indication of her resourcefulness, desperation, and hope.

The Genotti family is composed of the father Carlo, the mother Margherita, both in their mid-forties, Loretta (sixteen), Sophia (fifteen), Maria (thirteen), and two younger children who were not present at the interview.

MINUCHIN: First, I want to understand what has been happening. Loretta has been losing weight for the last three years. Is that correct?

LORETTA: Right.

Note: A different analysis of this interview appears in Minuchin, Rosman, and Baker, *Psychosomatic Families.* A videotape of the session which may be used for professional training purposes is available from the South Beach Psychiatric Center, Staten Island, New York.

FATHER: Two years.

M: When did it start, Loretta?

FATHER: Two years.

MOTHER: It started at the beginning of Lent. I take her to St. Francis Hospital because Loretta, she don't feel too good. She got pain all over. So they want to take picture inside Loretta's stomach, but I say no. I say, "I take my daughter home."

M: Do you remember that, Loretta? (*She nods.*)

MOTHER: So I take Loretta home because I don't want nobody to touch my daughter. So I take her home, and next day Loretta throws up. She cries. She has a pain. So I call the car service, put Loretta in the car, and take her to Dr. Smith. He calls Tenafly Hospital, and from there we go straight to Tenafly Hospital. Loretta stay in bed two weeks there in the hospital.

M: From your point of view, Loretta, what was it that you were having?

I am listening to what the family is saying, but I am triggered by the parents' persistence in replying to questions posed to Loretta. I know from previous experience that Loretta's symptoms may be expected to improve as she begins to gain the autonomy proper to a sixteen-year-old. I also know that Loretta's dependency and her mother's concern are interacting elements of the same pattern: whenever I touch one, I will touch the other.

LORETTA: The first night I went to St. Francis Hospital was because I was having strong pains in my abdomen and my back, and they found it was a kidney infection so they gave me intravenous since the pain was so great.

M: Okay, so you went then for something very specific. And when you went to the Tenafly Hospital, was it a continuation of the same?

LORETTA: I don't know. I mean, they never actually said anything there.

M: Since your mother is the memory of the family, she can tell, but you'll need to check it because it's your life that she's describing. Okay?

The mother is clearly the most powerful member of the family, at least in relation to anything involving Loretta's illness. Everything demands that I respect that—the mother's real power, the rules of courtesy, and the necessity of maintaining enough observance of the family's accustomed patterns to join them in a therapeutic system. At the same time, I begin to signal the message that will dominate the session: Loretta should possess her own experience.

MOTHER: So I take her to Tenafly to my doctor. For two weeks they check Loretta. Loretta, she doesn't eat enough, and the doctor told me, "Take your daughter home and bring her to a psychiatrist."

M: Hold it a moment—I want to check something. Loretta, when you were in the hospital, you didn't eat anything?

LORETTA: For a while they put a sign up on my bed that said I wasn't supposed to eat anything because they didn't know what was causing the pain. And then I didn't have any appetite. So I had the IVs from the first time until I went home.

M: Do you know that this happens to many people? If they go two or three days without eating, they lose their appetite. It was at this point that you stopped eating, and this was when? Two years ago?

Loretta has responded to my attention, and my polite indication that her mother isn't the ultimate authority, with increased information—a good sign. My statement begins to normalize her experience, one way of challenging her position as the sick member of the family.

LORETTA: Right.

MOTHER: So I stay two weeks with Loretta in the hospital.

M: You stayed in the hospital? *With* her?

My tone of voice conveys genuine admiration for this woman, who rode roughshod over the bureaucracy of an entire city hospital.

FATHER: Yes, she spent many nights with her.

M: That's wonderful. That's an Italian heart for you!

MOTHER: One day, my husband told me to come home to see the kids and said, "If you still want to go tomorrow, I'll take you in there." So I said I would see what I can do. So we go home. When I go home, I got a funny feeling. Loretta, she doesn't feel good, so I say to my husband, "You better take me back to the hospital. I have a funny feeling about Loretta." He say, "Oh no, you stay here." I say, "You take me or I go." So my husband take me there. When I go back, I find Loretta all black and blue. She has pains. She's screaming, "I have a pain all over here, I have a pain over there!" She is screaming. I say, "We will call the doctor." So they say nothing is wrong with Loretta. And I say, "What do you mean nothing is wrong with Loretta? She's all black and blue." "That's all right, don't get nervous." So they give her needle, and Loretta, she sleep all night.

M: That means, you had the feeling—

MOTHER: Loretta could die.

I have a problem. It is clear that Mrs. Genotti's and Loretta's overinvolvement with each other is dysfunctional. But it is also clear that this is an accepted pattern in this family, buttressed by all the power of the Mama in Sicilian culture. I am going to have to find a way of challenging the overinvolvement while accepting the Genottis' norms.

M: Do you have the same sense about your daughter Maria?

MOTHER: Yes, with everybody. All my kids.

M: I don't think Maria sends vibes. What do you think, Maria? If you have a pain, do you think Mama knows?

MARIA: Yes.

M: She does! What about your father? That's a special gift. Does he have that?

MARIA: Yes.

M: Is that so, Carlo? Can you experience the pain of your kids as your wife does?

FATHER: Well, I can see by just taking a look at them. If they don't look good, then I assume there's something wrong, you know.

M: But Margherita says she can hear vibrations from the hospital.

FATHER: I brought her back from the hospital, right? The minute that we were home, she says, "I want to go back." When she got back, Loretta was in bad shape.

The father claims no magical knowledge of his children's well-being, but he makes it clear that he has no intention of challenging his wife's claims. Now I know—if I didn't before—that I can't challenge Mama or motherhood in this family. But perhaps I can challenge its definition.

M: That feeling is very, very important when the kids are young. That's essential. Let me ask you a little bit, Loretta. You are sixteen now?

LORETTA: Yes.

M: Now that you're growing up, does it sometimes bother you that Mama is still so sensitive to you?

LORETTA: Sometimes.

M: Sophia, what's your feeling? Sometimes she forgets you're fifteen? Treats you as if you were younger?

SOPHIA: Yes.

M: This always happens. When you are very sensitive to the pains of younger kids, there is then a problem of how to become the mother of older children. A good mother of younger children sometimes becomes a difficult mother for older children. So you are still a very good mother for Maria, Giuseppi, and Enrico, but I think there is some problem with Sophia and Loretta. I think you're too much for them!

MOTHER: No. (*Father laughs.*) How?

I have been with the Genottis for thirty minutes, immersed in their experience, absorbing their language, observing their transactions. With their help, I have begun to compose a therapeutic theme that will become the arena in which I'll challenge their reality. Replacing "we are a normal family with an anorectic child and helpful parents," the therapeutic exploration will follow the theme, "You are a family that got stuck in your development and must grow up to adjust to the growth of your adolescent children." The family and I will build this alternative with material carefully culled from their own language and transactions, so that they can feel they are still dealing with the familiar. As the session continues, the alternative will make it possible to challenge the rigidity of this family organization and to free Loretta from her role as family stabilizer.

LORETTA: You always have arguments with me and Sophia. Always.

M: Carlo, help the two girls to talk, because Mama is too strong and they're in the hot spot. Help them to say how they would like Mama to be sometimes.

FATHER: Why don't you express yourselves about what the doctor is saying? At fifteen, you should know how to say a few words by yourself, huh?

SOPHIA: I don't have too many fights with Mom.

FATHER: We're talking about how you wish Mama treats you from now on, since you have become fifteen.

SOPHIA: I don't know. She doesn't treat me bad.

Sophia is already retreating; clearly no one in this family is comfortable challenging the mother.

FATHER: Do you think Mama needs to be changed to somehow make you feel better?

LORETTA: Dad, you really can't change. Once you are the person you are, you have to try, and compromise a little.

FATHER: But you wish that Mama could change toward you somehow.

LORETTA: I'm not saying change totally. I'd rather have her worry less.

M: What you're saying, Loretta, is that it's not a total change, but you would like your mother to be less worried about you and about the other kids.

LORETTA: M-hm.

It is not easy for Loretta and her father to talk. Carlo also has areas of Old World rigidity and protectiveness about his daughters' growing up. Furthermore, he experiences great difficulty in standing up to his wife. The girls cannot trust him to be an effective ally. I intervene by restating Loretta's challenge, softening it to a point that may be acceptable, and lending support to an agreement between Loretta and her father.

M: Do you think that Mama has too big a heart and that sometimes this makes her worry more than is necessary?

FATHER: Well, what I've seen, Mama does herself much of the things that the girls could do by themselves. She makes it too easy for them. Now they find it a little hard to begin to manage by themselves and try out new situations.

M: That's a very interesting and very sensitive view. Can you say it again? Because I think Margherita is deaf in this ear (*touches her ear*).

My carefully chosen adjectives make the father my peer: someone who understands the intricacies of psychological processes. At the same time, a slightly seductive, humorous gesture softens my challenge to his wife. I want these people to be able to talk to each other.

FATHER: I'm sure Margherita understood already what I'm talking about.

M: Do you understand what he says? What do you think about that?

MOTHER: Why do I have to think? I'm a mother. The things they can't do, I do.

M: If the kids say "Do something," you do?

MOTHER: What should I do—let the kids down?

M: Now, what about what Carlo says? That you do more than what they need.

FATHER: You've been doing, and you don't mind doing anything for them, right?

MOTHER: I don't. I help my kids all the time in all ways. If they want help, my kids, I give it to them. That's what I do for my kids, then, all the time.

M: I think you still did not hear clearly what your husband said, and what Loretta said. Say it again, Loretta, so that Margherita can hear it.

Margherita has a stone-wall defense: all she is doing is being a good mother. But now both Carlo and Loretta are prepared to challenge the overprotective pattern, especially since my bantering is establishing a lighter, more secure feeling. Now it is safe to do a little exploring.

LORETTA: You worry too much. And you've got to try to worry less, because I'm sixteen and Sophia is fifteen and Maria is thirteen and you worry too much, as if we were ten and not sixteen or fifteen. And let us try to do some things by ourselves. Because if we want to try something, you say, "No, let me do it. It's better if I do it."

MOTHER: Wait a minute, Loretta, I give you the chance . . .

LORETTA: In certain things that are easy to do. But in other things, you don't dare give us a chance.

M: Loretta, I want to congratulate you! I think you're very good. Sophia, do you help her sometimes?

In my work with anorectics, I have observed that a capacity for direct challenge *in an area not related to food* is a prerequisite for improvement. So I strongly reward Loretta's competent statement while beginning to explore the possibility of gathering support for her by strengthening her position as leader of the sibling subsystem.

SOPHIA: Help in what?

M: Do you help Loretta? Because she took the leadership position to defend all three of you. Do you sometimes join her?

SOPHIA: No.

M: So, Loretta, you're the only fighter?

LORETTA: Yes.

M: Carlo, you have a lovely wife. Your children have a lovely mother. But I think she can become a problem for the children who are growing up.

FATHER: Yes, I thought that too. In the situation of these two girls, now that they wish to do things but they are not really prepared to do, just because . . .

M: They didn't have any experience. Yes.

LORETTA: Yes. But there has to be some point where you begin.

FATHER: And that causes more worry for my wife, you know, when the two girls are willing to do something we might consider unusual.

M: What kind of things? I'm interested in your point of view.

FATHER: Say Sophia wants to go out at night. My wife will decide whether or not to let her go out.

SOPHIA (*laughing*): I think it's the other way around.

MOTHER: I think so too. I'm sorry. I don't agree with that.

FATHER: You think it's the other way too? Who's most worried, me or Mama?

SOPHIA: Oh, she's worried about it, but she's willing to let us go, while you're—you know.

MOTHER: Thank you, Sophia. Thank God!

FATHER: What I wanted to say is, she's the one who worries; she worries too much. So she might prefer not to let her go so she won't worry so much when at ten o'clock she hasn't come home yet.

It seems that overprotective patterns are triggered when the adolescent girls request more autonomy. It is possible that both mother and father react by controlling strongly, but that each perceives the other parent as the chief discipliner. There is another factor involved, since Loretta and Sophia attend an inner-city high school.

FATHER: You have to worry. If they went out and weren't back on time . . .

MOTHER: I'm a mother, right? So I say, "You have to watch yourself and at ten o'clock you have to be home." What's wrong with that?

M: I don't know that anything is wrong.

FATHER: You know, the news has been so bad. We don't want these kids getting into—you know. Drugs, and sex, and—

As a father I recognize and respect the parents' fear. The issue becomes how to accept parental protection and at the same time encourage the children's autonomy.

M: Loretta, can you disagree with your mother?

LORETTA: I can disagree, but it gets into an argument. Sometimes I don't even bother, because I know already that the situation is going to turn out to be an argument.

M: Can you disagree with your father?

LORETTA: No, neither one of them is easy, because if I disagree with one, then they get together and the two of them think one way.

M: Do you remember any specific situation in which you disagreed with them?

LORETTA: I can't think of one.

The session has shown that Loretta can enter successfully into interpersonal conflict, but it seems that her self-perception is that she will always lose. This is quite characteristic of the inner experience of anorectic girls, who grow up in an atmosphere in which conflicts are to be avoided, loyalty toward others encourages accommodation, and to disagree is a betrayal of the family value system.

M: What about you, Sophia? Can you disagree with Mom?

SOPHIA: No.

M: Can you disagree with Dad?

SOPHIA: I don't think so.

LORETTA: You do once in a while, though, Sophia.

M: But you think you can't. Okay. What about you, Maria, can you disagree with Mom?

MARIA: Not really. She always wins.

M: She always wins. And what about Dad? Can you disagree with him? (*Maria sighs.*) Sophia, let's say you want something very strongly. Can you convince your mother?

By exploring the experiences of the three teenagers and emphasizing their similarities as subsystem members, I am decentralizing Loretta as a patient.

SOPHIA: I don't think so.

M: The girls feel that you are too strong for them.

MOTHER: No.

M: They said yes.

MOTHER: With Sophia, there are no problems. She never asks me anything on which I have to say yes or no. We have a little problem with Loretta.

M: Margherita, you're not hearing.

LORETTA: I'd like to interrupt for a minute. It's a big problem with my parents coming from the old country and us being raised and educated and born here, because we use certain words and they don't understand them.

MOTHER: Oh, Loretta.

LORETTA: Like right now, you're getting kind of angry because I'm saying this, but it's true. You don't understand sometimes what Daddy's saying or the doctor is saying or even what I'm saying now. You're getting angry with me.

Loretta came to the session depressed and desperately weary of being "the problem." Therapeutic interventions have restated the problem: negotiating rules for growing up. Loretta has picked the issue up and is stating it effectively.

Other themes have begun to appear: the anorectic's preoccupation with her appearance and her fear of growing fat; the parents' desperate sense that they are prisoners in an insane war over food and eating; Loretta's sense that she is an embattled, solitary, and doomed fighter. In each case, I try to keep the focus on the battle for control and the adolescent's natural striving for independence, expanding the theme to include the spouses' conflicts, the father's isolation from his daughters, and his inability to challenge his wife's behavior as a parent. Whenever possible, I make links between Carlo and Loretta: one way of introducing distance between the mother and the children is to support greater closeness between the father and Loretta. Now, an hour into the session, it is time for lunch.

M (*looks at watch*): It's 12:15. I want to have something to eat now. Loretta, I think you're a good fighter. I'm impressed by you.

FATHER: She is, yes.

M: But I'm concerned about what she feels. If she feels that she can't fight and win, then she will probably starve herself.

MOTHER: She is big enough to do anything she wants to do. Sophia, the same. (*The food, previously ordered by the family, is brought in. Loretta runs out of the room, crying that she will not eat. I go after her.*)

Having lunch with anorectic families makes it possible, in some cases, to move the spotlight from the anorectic's eating to the interpersonal family transactions that revolve around eating: control, obedience/disobedience, blackmail, and demands for loyalty. Sometimes the explicit enactment of these conflicts leads to crises that jolt the identified patient and the family out of their pathological patterns. In this case the mere appearance of food activated Loretta's usual obstinacy. The family, waiting in the therapy room, probably felt they were back to square one. But talking to Loretta in the hallway, I was able to build on her positive experience of the first part of the session. Loretta and I agreed that she was not going to eat; she was going to negotiate with her parents, and win. I promised to help, and she returned to the therapy room with that understanding. Meanwhile the mother had distributed sandwiches and drinks and had placed a sandwich next to Loretta's chair. As I sat down I said I had an agreement with Loretta that she was not going to eat in the session but that the rest of the family should have their lunch.

M: Loretta, how old does your mother think you are?
LORETTA: I don't know. Apparently not sixteen.
M: I absolutely agree with you. Until you are sixteen, you won't eat properly.
MOTHER: She wins me all the time, my daughter! If I say no, Loretta stops eating. If we don't do it Loretta's way, we have to hold our hands in the air, we have to stop everybody. I have to stop Sophia. I have to stop my husband. I have to stop the phone ring. I can't talk to nobody because Loretta, she nervous. She do anything to send me, my husband, her sister, her brothers, any way she wants. We say, "Yes, Loretta." We have to do anything she wants, and everything will be okay. If we do something else forget about it; Loretta, she say no.

(*As she talks, the rest of us begin to eat; as if by design we avoid looking in Loretta's direction.*)

M: Can you answer your mother, Loretta? Carlo, let Mama sit near Loretta. Loretta, talk with Mama because she says that you're controlling the house.

Although Loretta's feeling is one of being helplessly controlled, her control of her family in terms of food is second only to

Mama's control in terms of protection. But since psychosomatic families are conflict avoiders, all controlling maneuvers are put under the heading of concern and protection. The therapeutic challenge to this family pattern is to encourage explicit conflict in areas of normal autonomy.

LORETTA: I'm not controlling nobody, Mama.

MOTHER: You're controlling your father, you're controlling me, Sophia, Enrico, Maria, Giuseppi. Why, Loretta?

LORETTA: I'm not controlling nobody. It's just that somebody has to do something.

MOTHER: That's me and your father's job. You have to do something by yourself. You are not to interfere with Sophia, Maria . . .

LORETTA: I want to stand by myself and you're stopping me!

MOTHER: No, Loretta.

LORETTA: Yes, Mama! You may not realize this sometimes, but you're doing it anyway.

MOTHER: But sometimes, Loretta, you put us in the world in a way we can't do nothing. We have to agree with you. But sometimes we can't. And if you don't get what you want, you start crying.

LORETTA: No, Mama.

MOTHER: Screaming. Throwing chairs around. Pulling anything the way you want.

M: She has temper tantrums? Like little children?

Now conflict is in the open. I have supported Loretta's behavior as an appropriate resistance to her parents' overcontrol. So I can support her parents' challenge of her childish behavior and still be perceived as supporting her competence. This encourages both the open expression of conflicts and the reciprocal demands for more suitable behavior.

FATHER: Well, she's perfectly all right when she's cool. When she blow the cool—

M: You agree with your wife that Loretta is the one that drives the house?

LORETTA: That's not the truth! You're making me sound like a bad person!

MOTHER (*gently*): No, you're not a bad person.

Loretta has signaled discomfort with the level of conflict, and the mother, as always, has responded protectively. My job is to block the family's pattern of transforming issues of behavior control into emotional blackmail. So I keep the conflict going.

M: She's saying that you have temper tantrums, Loretta. She's saying that you're childish.

LORETTA: I may yell, I may scream. But I am not childish. I don't ever throw things around.

MOTHER: Loretta, I don't say that—

LORETTA: If anything, *you* throw shoes at me or whatever it is that's in your way. You're trying to make me sound like a bad person!

MOTHER: No, Loretta. You're not a bad person.

Again there has been a warning light and a response. But this time Loretta herself continues her point.

LORETTA: I'm the bad person in the family. I'm the black sheep of the family simply because I stand up and say what I feel. The other kids are always good. They're always your little sweethearts because they don't open their mouths.

MOTHER: No, Loretta, nobody is sweetheart . . .

LORETTA: They agree about everything with you and Daddy. Whatever you say is all right with them.

MOTHER: When you want something I can't buy you, you cry for three days, you get nervous. You stop eating. Right away—no food. Not get up from the bed. You don't want to see nobody. You don't want to talk to nobody. And Mama cries.

M: Is your mother saying that you're blackmailing them? That your not eating is a way of controlling them?

Loretta and Margherita are involved in an interesting pas de deux. Following my lead, they began a tentative exploration of direct disagreement. That necessitates distancing, but distancing appears to make them uncomfortable. Both respond with guilt-producing statements ("You're calling me a bad person"; "You're a blackmailer who makes me suffer") that will facilitate closeness. Luckily, the mother's statement can be used to tie Loretta's symptom to family functioning, transforming her not eating into an interpersonal transaction. This reframing can move the symptom away from Loretta's body, into the hands of all the family members.

LORETTA: That's not true!
MOTHER: So you do the same thing to the hospital! You black-mail the doctor.
LORETTA: I don't blackmail nobody.
MOTHER: That's what they told me. You don't eat. They bring food in and you give it to somebody else.
LORETTA: It always turns out that I'm the liar.

Now both the mother and I have firmly labeled not eating as a manipulative act. But as often happens, the facts of the matter are quickly transformed into the emotional interchanges of mother and daughter: "You didn't eat in the hospital" flipflops with "You don't trust me."

MOTHER: Now, you have to tell Dr. Minuchin you stay almost two months with no food in the stomach. Only that kind of food they give you through the tube. You cry. Mama cries out-side in the hallway when they put the tube in the nose. Mama cries.
LORETTA: I'm not going to feel sorry for you, Ma. I'm sorry be-cause you're wrong. I am not a liar.
MOTHER: You made a cake for me to eat, I don't want to eat it. You right away say, "You don't want to eat it because I made it." The doctor at the hospital told me, "Your daughter is in danger and could die." I see she don't eat nothing. Now, this morning, she get up and she come over here. Not even a glass of water. There's nothing in there. I have to worry about her.

We are firmly back in the endless fight about eating. I want to reintroduce an interpersonal perspective.

M: I think Loretta feels like a loser in your family. You say Loretta is a winner. I think she's a loser.

MOTHER: I can't do anything with Loretta. Loretta says, "You don't love me because you don't want to get this," and I have to do what Loretta say.

M: I don't think you let her feel that she is sixteen.

MOTHER: No, she is the winner. Loretta, Mama don't tell you you are sixteen?

LORETTA: Yeah, you tell me, but you don't make me feel it. You don't treat me like sixteen. You treat me like I was two years old.

Loretta is using my developmental construction as a crutch to help her stand up against her mother.

M: Margherita, you do so many things for your daughter that she becomes an extremely childish, incompetent person.

FATHER: Right. I have to agree with you.

M: And at some point your daughter needs to grow up. And your wife needs to start to grow up first, so that your daughter can grow up. It's very difficult, Loretta, to fight your mother because she is a very lovely mother. Carlo, how can you help your daughter to become sixteen? Because she will begin to eat only when she really is sixteen, not before.

FATHER: I wish she'd make clear to me what she wants to do. I wish she'd be reasonable and understand that sometimes things are not possible.

M: You know, Loretta is very childish. But I think the family, and particularly you, Margherita, support her childishness.

MOTHER: How? How, Loretta?

M: When you tell her *how* to move the chair, you're treating her as if she's six. That's how. It's very simple how. When you tell her that she can go out with a boyfriend without asking her father because you will protect her from her father's anger, that's how. You keep her as a little child.

I have labeled a family member ("Loretta, you are childish") and at the same time assigned responsibility for that label to another ("Margherita, you keep her childish"). It is a framing that suggests a solution: "Loretta is childish; therefore, Margherita must grow up."

FATHER: When the tempers rise between the two of them, it's not possible to understand Loretta. Most of the time, even a little thing creates a situation that becomes impossible because of tempers.

M: I think you need to talk to your wife about keeping Loretta a little girl.

FATHER: I'll be yelling many times that she's doing just too much and won't let these girls do things they could do. Even when they were younger. And I don't think much has changed in that area.

M: Can Margherita hear you, or is she deaf?

MOTHER: No, I hear my husband. I hear what he say. But I want to tell you something. Loretta, she grew up a long time ago. When she wants to be, she's a young teenager. She knows it.

M: No, Loretta, I don't think you're a grown-up person. I think you're very much tied to your mother, unable to make decisions, to take initiative. You're fighting a battle for growing up in the worst possible way—killing yourself so that you will demonstrate to Mama that she is wrong. I think you can be a winner, but I don't know yet that you want to. You will eat only when you are sixteen. But I don't think you feel, act, or think like sixteen. And I think this is because the family, especially Mama, is always doing things for you. Mother is moving your hands; she is moving your arms. (*I take Loretta's hands and arms and move them.*) You don't have anything that's your own. So I think you shouldn't eat now. But you will eat at the moment you become sixteen.

My behavior, treating Loretta like a puppet, has focused her attention on me; it increases her distance from her mother. At the same time, by appropriating Loretta's control of the symptom ("you will eat only when you are sixteen") I have removed its metaphorical meaning as a banner of autonomy. Not eating is framed as a symbol of Loretta's *dependence;* and since I have joined with Loretta in her struggle for autonomy, we are now cooperating to create a family context that will allow her to eat and grow.

In effect, *we* are struggling for family change. Within this framing, I negotiate an agreement with Loretta. She will eat—but she will eat alone, away from the family table. I will weigh her when she comes to sessions, but her weight will remain a secret between her and me. With this agreed on, I move toward the end of the session by introducing the focus on eating reframed as an issue of autonomy.

M: Loretta, I think you should not start eating with the family until you're sixteen. How old are you now?

LORETTA: Sixteen.

M: When was your birthday?

LORETTA: Last week.

M: But you're not sixteen yet. And since Loretta will not start eating until she is sixteen, I want Loretta to eat alone. At the point when she begins to eat, she will be exactly sixteen. I think, Loretta, that you should not put too much weight on because your face looks rather nice long. But you need to gain probably ten pounds. This is for you to decide. Because at sixteen, you will need to do things on your own. At home I want you, Carlo, to talk with your wife, and then talk with Loretta, about what rights a sixteen-year-old has and what obligations. Can you help your wife to think like that? That a sixteen-year-old has obligations?

FATHER: I will try.

M: Can she hear?

MOTHER: I hear good.

M: Okay. Carlo, you'll need to talk with Margherita. I think she has run the house for too long alone, you know. You'll need to talk with your father about jobs, Loretta. Maybe he can help you with this and other things. Carlo, can you begin to let Loretta know you . . .

FATHER: What I want for Loretta—excuse me for interrupting you—is to think different about me. She has to think about me not as an obstacle course.

LORETTA: Well, I can't think it, Dad, unless you show it.

M: In this week I want you, Loretta, to talk to your father twice for half an hour. Maybe the first time you tell him something about you, okay? So that he'll know you. The second time, I want you to tell her something about yourself, Carlo. I think she needs to know you, and that will be a help. Carlo should take over more of helping Loretta. Will that be a help, Margherita? Margherita, she'll start eating when she's sixteen, and she won't die of that. If she loses weight, then we'll think differently. If she maintains the weight she has now, it's safe for the moment. So don't worry about that.

The family left in a mood of hope, with a new and more productive definition of their problems. I had lived with them for two hours. In the "condensed time" of a therapeutic session, transactions have an experiential intensity that permits a holistic vision. I knew this family's strength, their flexibility, and their capacity to increase their behavioral repertory. I felt that Loretta had already begun to change, and I had seen Carlo and Margherita expand their repertories in their transactions with me. My prognosis for the Genotti family was positive.

They continued in treatment for four months. Therapy focused on issues of individuation and independence. Loretta gained 21 pounds over the first three months; her weight stabilized at around 105 pounds. A follow-up one and a half years later found Loretta working as a waitress, a job she had held for the last six months. She had reenrolled in high school and was planning to finish. She had many friends and maintained a stormy relationship with her parents.

AUTHOR: Any questions?

READER: No, I don't have any questions.

AUTHOR: That presents a problem. If you don't function as an unconvinced reader, I can't function as a convincing author.

READER: Are you so dependent?

AUTHOR: That's an interesting word. I presume you are using it to describe my character. But how can you have a single dependent person?

READER: I know many dependent people, including myself.

AUTHOR: Then you understand my point. Humans are dependent by definition. We interdepend because we are parts. Do you think Margherita is dependent?

READER: Well, she is larger than life. The way she picks up vibes from the family ... yes, she is dependent, but in a different way. She depends on the children's being dependent on her. That is, well, now wait a minute—

AUTHOR: Words are mere carriers. We should be able to control them instead of the other way around. Loretta and Margherita are interdependent. But when we try to describe their interactions, we have too many short phrases. We dichotomize to clarify—white/black, dependent/independent. Brief either/ors and cause/effects make matters beautifully clear. But life doesn't oblige. It continues to be complex, unclear, a Pandora's box of mud.

READER: Do I detect hostility? I thought the relationship between author and reader should be one of intellectual harmony.

AUTHOR: Sorry. I've learned to recoil from logical simplification. To describe life we need metaphors; objectivity will not suffice.

READER: But don't we need frameworks? Models, ways of describing?

AUTHOR: I remember a book by Papini in which a sculptor in search of the creative moment was sculpting a wax figure with red hot chisels. The figure was destroyed at the moment of construction.

READER: What does that have to do with families?

AUTHOR: Nothing. But it has to do with traps. I want to describe a family dance, in which individuals are dancers, dance, and music.

READER: Yeats? Would you mind if we got away from poetry and back to my questions?

AUTHOR: What are your questions?

READER: Okay. I accept that you had good results with the Genottis and with anorexia. But I have doubts about the benefits of your approach for the individual family member.

AUTHOR: I would have been concerned if you'd had certainties. Doubts are avenues to questions and, with luck, to the acceptance of uncertainty. What troubles you?

READER: Loretta, Margherita, Sophia, Carlo, Maria ... What is the impact of family therapy on each one of them? In individual therapy, growth evolves through the experiential encounter between therapist and patient, and through the exploration of early experiences in a context of respect and mutual acceptance. Is that correct?

AUTHOR: For our dialog, it may suffice. Where are your questions leading us?

READER: Why should the Genotti individuals change?

AUTHOR: That is the Gordian knot. Should I cut it or unravel it for you?

READER: I will accept any metaphor that helps me understand.

AUTHOR: Okay. The road may be long and meandering. We start with the Genottis a year ago when Loretta developed her symptoms. We make the assumption that up to this point the family lived in a more or less predictable environment and was a more or less functional family. With Loretta and Sophia entering adolescence and the adolescent world, their demands challenged the family's implicit organizational structure, and the Genottis' reliance on loyalty and interdependency was challenged by Loretta's and Sophia's forays into the outside world. Now—and this is an interesting paradox—Loretta developed a symptom of rebellion that also contained increased closeness. It was change without changing, since her illness elicited a concern and overcontrol common in this family, while her rebellion was confined to food. It's what systems analysts call a first-order change: the individual changes in a way that maintains the system's patterns.

READER: When the Genottis came to you, what were your goals?

AUTHOR: Always in cases of anorexia, cure and growth, in that order. But because Loretta was in no immediate physical danger, my interventions with the Genottis could be based on the complementarity of growth and cure. My interventions were for the most part directed to challenging the family's rigidity and giving family members the experience of an expanded reality. Let's look back at the session. At the beginning of the interview I observed Mother/Loretta operating at a level of proximity that had built—I assumed—over time, until they had all the mobility of flies in molasses. This interpersonal context controlled their view of themselves and the others, determined in great measure their affective range, and was maintained by the language and actions they shared. Of course their relationship contained and was contained by the larger system of the family. But let's focus on Loretta for a moment, since you are curious about the way family therapy impinges on the individual. Loretta's experience of herself was the experience of self in context. In the family, the contexts are the other members in a predictable organization. The Loretta/Mother dyad had certain patterns. But when I joined them, supporting Loretta's right to challenge, the pattern changed and so did her experience and language. When I supported Carlo, validating his voice, and he challenged Margherita's overinvolvement with her daughters, Loretta, from the perspective of a sibling, got a different experience of self and other. The same occurred when she experimented with challenging her parents as the oldest daughter, when she felt betrayed by Sophia, when I supported Margherita in her challenge of Loretta's exploitation, when Carlo asked her for understanding, when her symptoms were tied to the family, and so on. Loretta, like a piece in a kaleidoscope, experiences herself in different configurations—central or peripheral, brilliant or opaque, large or small, foreground or background, and in each position she is circling around herself, experiencing new movements, new distances, new intensities, new silences, new words. And as her view of the other family members changed, as they exhibited more facets than they had previously shown, transformation of meaning also went on in the other Genottis. Not the same meaning, not at the same time. Tension was experienced among them, since they were impinged upon by uncertainty from different perspectives. The world was no longer predictable. And as the Genottis, like you and me, need coherence and meaning, a search for meaning developed. I was there with new metaphors, descriptions, reframings. Since we are creatures of redundance, the Genottis repeated these new patterns between different members, with different contents, and at successive times. As this happens, old sets begin to break up. With any luck at all, the Genottis begin to experience themselves and each other as more complex. They are people with differences, who have more than one way of responding.

READER: But is this enough? Don't they have to understand where they're coming from? Don't you believe in the significance of childhood experience and the power of experiential models to organize the individual's behavior?

AUTHOR: If I say yes, I will dilute my message. If I say no, I will dilute my message. I can't go on.

READER: If you can't go on, please continue.

Part Two

Patterns of Violence

"Mata a su madre sin causa justificada" (He killed his mother without justification). Clearly the killing of a mother was not news to this New York City Spanish newspaper. The lure to the reader was the "lack of justification." As a student of family process I am well acquainted with the emotions that permeate family transactions: rage, frustration, helplessness, envy, protectiveness, love, concern. The people closest to us become the recipients of our emotional gifts and confusions, and we are their projection screens as they are ours. The cauldron of emotions shapes family members into beings who are not always predictable, not always logical or rational, not always in control of their responses.

But violence, or the implementation of emotional transactions in a destructive channel, is something else. To understand that, we have to look beyond the family. Family violence requires a frame that is semipermeable, so that the blood and tears flow in and out of the picture. Such a frame can be found in the headlines of any daily paper.

VIOLENCE HITS MIAMI A THIRD DAY
TALKS IN ISRAEL FAIL
EL SALVADOR SAYS 12% OF TROOPS KILLED OR HURT
ARGENTINES TRY TO FORGET THE FALKLANDS CONFLICT
UNEMPLOYMENT AT 10%

This selection from the *Philadelphia Inquirer* of December 31, 1982, does not include the riots in India, bombings in Manila, Johannesburg, Ireland, and England, acid rain, the increase of soup kitchens needed by the hungry in the United States, or continuing famine in the Third World. For that, one had to await the evening news. Within this cauldron, the mental-health and legal systems are charged with monitoring and stabilizing family violence. Their approach has generally been to focus on the family as an independent unit. But looking at the family apart from its social context is like studying the dynamics of swimming by examining a fish in a frying pan. The result is intervention without perspective.

In my professional life, my most prolonged institutional contact with family violence was as a child psychiatrist at the Wiltwyck School for Boys. It was a time of creativity for me, but I know now that my involvement in the process also distorted my perceptions; while I was expanding the therapeutic field I was also maintaining the structure of the system I was challenging.

Wiltwyck was a private nonprofit residential treatment center for one hundred boys, eight to twelve years of age. These children were the products of slums.

> They have rolled drunks and interchanged with pimps, prostitutes and addicts in their hallways or on the crowded, smelly stoops. These children live in dire poverty; they have seen alcoholism, homosexuality, addiction, promiscuity, prostitution, and mental illness. Much is in their own families. Pathology and poverty have seeped into their lives with such a pervasive dark insistence that many of them know of no other existence or reality. This *is* reality. You fend for yourself. If there is no food at home, you steal—from your neighbor, cousin or local shopkeeper. If you're lucky enough to steal money that's even better. You don't have to be home at any hour. Meal times are vague. And home may be some space in a bed with other kids. In the summer you pour out on the dirty streets and look for action and excitement. You keep moving and roaming and running. And you do things. Because when there is excitement and motion you can finally experience yourself as *somebody*.

These children were referred to the school, for the most part, by the Juvenile Court with the label of "delinquent or neglected juvenile." It seemed clear to me then that the delinquent act requires a social focus. I rebelled against the narrow frame of the juridical system and began a study of the families of these children. My team (Edgar H. Auerswald, Charles King, Braulio Montalvo,

Clara Rabinowitz) and I became interested in the patterns of communication among family members: the disjointed manner of dialog, with members talking at each other, and the strong inter-personal component, where two plus two might or might not equal four, depending on your relation with the other. And of course we studied control and the quality of all-or-nothing that characterized parental responses to children's misbehavior. There was at times no response and at others an uncontrolled barrage that passed as appropriate punishment. There was violence from parents to children, from children to children, and frequently from children to parents. The social context of these families, at the socioeconomic margin of society, trickled down into their daily reality as a heavy fog of hopelessness. We were nonetheless impressed by the untapped resources of the family members, and we developed family interventions designed to help them use their own bootstraps to pull themselves up. Knowing the weakness of mental-health interventions in the sociopolitical arena, we re-stricted our efforts to the development of therapeutic techniques for working with these families.

On the strength of this work, I became Professor of Child Psy-chiatry at the University of Pennsylvania. It never occurred to me then to question the procedures by which children were plucked out of their families and placed in the institution. I accepted the court's knowledge of norms and its legal right to determine and punish deviance. I was critical of individual judges but accepted the intention of the system to protect the children. I questioned but never challenged the procedures of the social worker for studying the family of the child: the uninvited home visit, often in the evening or at dinner time; the looking at the furniture, the pot in the oven, the contents of the refrigerator, and the general de-gree of cleanliness in the home; the questioning of the neighbors. Though I would never accept such intrusions into my own home, I accepted the procedures as necessary "in the best interests of the child." It was only later that I realized such intrusions were not only offensive but irrelevant; the delinquent act is not a direct consequence of these facets of family life, though society often as-sumes a connection.

Our therapeutic interventions were also more accepting of the juridical system than we realized. Though I challenged my colleagues' narrow concept of the psychological field and focused on the child as part of the family system, I drew boundaries that separated the family from its context. In staking my territory and proclaiming expertise on the interior of the family, I was declaring ignorance about other aspects of the family reality. By the process of dividing territory, I felt competent in *my* arena and supported the expertise of others in *their* field. I absolved myself of responsibility for the plight of the family until the moment of our encounter. In my view, I was brought in as an expert at the end of a chain of unfortunate events to mend what life and other people had pilfered and abused. The fault resides, I said in my internal monologs, in social and economic injustice; I am not part of the process of classifying, interpreting, and punishing these families. My expertise lies only in helping family members expand the range of their possibilities.

This process of parceling territory is essentially sound in a complex world where there is no place for the generalist. Yet as specialties have mushroomed, the result has been a skewing of reality. Each area deepens knowledge within its boundaries and develops specialized norms, but when all the exquisitely crafted pieces are put together, the whole is violated. Consider this United States Department of Health, Education, and Welfare statement about the number of professionals required to help families in which child abuse or neglect has occurred: "The abuse and neglect of children is a problem that cannot be managed by one discipline alone. A single case may involve social workers from both a hospital and the public child protection agency, a public assistance caseworker, one or more doctors, a psychiatrist or psychologist, both hospital and public health nurses, police, lawyers, a juvenile or family court judge, the child's school teacher, and any of a number of professionals." Eleven different institutions, without counting the family therapist, claim expertise about some part of the family body and, of course, challenge the expertise of anybody else who enters their territory. The statement frames the quandary in which members of the field find themselves; in order to function we need to specialize, but when we specialize we chop the ecology. Then what is the message? It seems to be:

(1) As human beings we belong to our culture and see what is

merely familiar as if it were the truth. One observes, studies, and intervenes in families and labels and punishes deviancy according to particular visions of appropriateness. Since the western world defends the rights of the individual, and the mental-health and juridical system are specially charged to protect children, it is possible to justify removal of the child to an institution.

(2) Professionals belong to systems with shared beliefs. They read the same journals and write papers for each other. As they explore their grain of sand, it increases in complexity, expands, and fills with time. It becomes their world. But professionals are proud and independent people. So psychiatrists and psychologists and social workers resent the idea that, as members of large social systems, they are charged by society with responsibility for monitoring and controlling deviance. They insist they are islanders. They see that psychiatric diagnoses have social purposes, but only vaguely. They participate in the juridical process that violates the family, but they don't see themselves participating.

(3) Social systems, like families, tend to maintain their organization unchanged. But since they are open systems, they also respond to inputs by restructuring. The challenge, then, is how to become an irritant for positive change. Mental-health professionals are programmed for certain social functions, but they can change the manner and even the meaning of their function.

As part of my education, I went to a family court in London. There I observed how violence was inflicted on the family by decent people charged to protect it. I reproduce my day in court here.

Family Dismemberment

A Day in Court

Three magistrates sit in the front of the room. The head magistrate is a man in his sixties. He seems warm and open, with an easy smile. Something about him makes me think he might be Jewish; I feel disposed to like him. His colleagues are an Indian man in his fifties and a woman in her forties. The man, dressed in impeccable British style, seems aloof—hiding behind his cultivated manner. The woman, blond and clearly Anglo-Saxon, sits on the edge of her chair, her body pushed forward in an attitude of curious contact with the plaintiffs. At their left, between the bench and the accused box, sits an usher in her twenties, dressed in an anonymity that blends perfectly with her desk. To the right stands the clerk, a West Indian lawyer in his late thirties. I decide that he mixes the formality of the court and the calypso rhythms of his own culture with ease. The court seems a wonderful kaleidoscope of the multiethnicity of London.

Two men who look like typical lawyers enter and present themselves to the clerk and then to the magistrates. Both are dressed in striped blue woolen suits, with striped ties. Both look English and are in their thirties. They smile as they identify themselves. Only later, when the proceedings have begun and it is possible to hear them talk for some time, do I realize that they don't speak real English at all. Theirs is a universal but sterile weaving of clichés and disconnected labels. They live in a world in which Paragraph G, Section A, clearly indicates a violation of Section D of Article 52.

The lawyers open their briefcases in synchrony and take out the instruments of their trade—typewritten pages of truncated lives, forcibly flattened to fit the 6″ x 12″ legal paper. They handle the paper with respect, as if it were possible, by legal alchemy, to reverse the process and squeeze restored lives out of these briefs.

I am a stranger here, a foreigner, and not only to London. Though I am wearing my professional face, it is human processes that interest me. The court is a world concerned with weighing and judging claims, assessing blame, and dispensing "justice." How does Paragraph G, Section A, apply to the intensely human concerns of a family court?

The clerk takes a folder from a social worker and hands it to the head magistrate. The three judges bend over it, conferring in low tones. The social worker gives a friendly nod to a young couple in the front row, and I stare at them curiously, realizing that this must be their case. They seem very young, mid-twenties at most. They are almost painfully well-groomed, obviously dressed in their Sunday best. Their clothing has been carefully pressed, but it is not of the highest quality. Actually the best-dressed member of the family is the baby, an active, smiling infant. She squirms in her mother's lap, trying to take her glasses. She moves her head back, holding the baby's hands, then rubs noses with her. The baby giggles.

The social worker is speaking. His report, he says, recommends that this child remain "in care" with the parents. The lawyer and magistrate leaf through the report. The couple tenses. The father takes the baby, who begins to pull his moustache. The magistrates confer in low voices, exchange comments with the lawyers. Then the magistrate announces that the court agrees with the social worker; the baby will remain in care with the parents. They rise and rush out, beaming. I don't understand, so I ask a visitor seated near me if he knows the family. He nods. What's the problem? That infant is this couple's second child, he tells me. The first was killed—smothered—at the age of six months by the mother, who "just couldn't make him stop crying." The mother was convicted of manslaughter with extenuating circumstances and served a jail sentence of two years. "This baby is five months old now," the man explains. The question is, should the court remove her? Or wait and see?

I don't envy those magistrates. This is the type of dilemma that they face in every case, the dilemma that all these social artifacts, including the court itself, cannot resolve. The court constantly has to decide between two evils. If it decides incorrectly, we may have to live with the death of a child. If it decides to remove a child, we must live with the responsibility of dismembering a family. The court feels no sure way of predicting. And the magistrates' only options are taking the child into custody or leaving her in the family where she is endangered. In the court structure, there are no options of intervening in the organization of the family as a support system. Either the child remains in the family, where she will live or die, or the child is removed from the family, to the hazards of foster care or a life in institutional care. Neither of these options is particularly attractive to the judges, who are committed and responsible people.

Probably the most frequently chosen option is "prevention." Which means—what? The second case is called.

Mrs. Obutu

As the clerk calls her name, an ample woman in her late thirties enters. She is dressed in a long, colorful African dress, with a kerchief around her head, carrying a one-year-old girl in her arms. Sylvia also enters: a fourteen-year-old, tall and thin, dressed in frayed jeans with the name of the designer claiming possession of one buttock. They come toward the magistrates, knowing that they will be participating in a ritual in which their destiny will be molded by foreign gods. There is a passivity in bodies imprinted by centuries of living in contexts that do not speak to them. I have a feeling that everyone is just repeating an ancestral dance; but clearly this is not so. Their dances are very different.

The lawyer representing the St. Vincent Borough presents the case to the magistrates; bracketed in his professional slang, the paragraphs, sections, and articles stand at attention. He then calls Sylvia's social worker to come to the box.

LAWYER: Please state your name and profession.
SOCIAL WORKER: Lucy Bennett. I am a social worker, working in Vincent Council.
LAWYER: Can you tell us what you know about the situation of Sylvia Obutu?

The atmosphere is friendly, relaxed, clearly that of two colleagues collaborating on a case.

SOCIAL WORKER: On the 12th of October I received a call from the 28th Precinct of the St. Vincent Borough telling me that they had a minor who had run away from home and refused to go back. I asked the police to bring the girl to my office and had a long conversation with her. Sylvia told me that her mother had beaten her and she was afraid of returning home. I asked her if the mother hit her or beat her, and if she understood the difference. She said that her mother had beat her with a stick and, at another time, with a shoe.

LAWYER: Did you try to convince her that she should return home?

SOCIAL WORKER: Yes, but she was too frightened.

LAWYER: What did you do?

SOCIAL WORKER: I obtained a safety order from the court and arranged for Sylvia to stay in St. Elizabeth Children's Home where she has been for the last two months.

2ND LAWYER: Did you make a home visit to Sylvia's home?

SOCIAL WORKER: Yes, I went and talked with Mrs. Obutu.

2ND LAWYER: Did you also talk with Mr. Obutu?

SOCIAL WORKER: No, he is now back in Ghana.

HEAD MAGISTRATE (to Mrs. Obutu): Do you want to say something now?

MRS. OBUTU: I want you to give me my daughter. She is *my* daughter!

CLERK (interrupting, to Mrs. Obutu): That's not the question.

HEAD MAGISTRATE (friendly): It's all right. I understand your wishes, Mrs. Obutu, and later when you go to the box, you can say that. But what I was asking you now is if you have anything to say or to ask Mrs. Bennett.

MRS. OBUTU: No.

The social worker steps down from the box, and Mrs. Obutu is called to testify. Now I begin to understand the structure of the judicial drama. One lawyer is defending the rights of Sylvia, a minor; the other represents the council. The social worker is Sylvia's social worker and is testifying for the council. All three are concerned in defending the "best interest of the child." Mrs.

Obutu, born in Ghana, with her African garb, her faulty English, and her one-year-old infant in her lap, doesn't have a chance. She is a chip in the kaleidoscope—a lonely red square in a yellow plane. This is, but is not, a criminal court. The magistrates are, but are not, judges; the two lawyers who defend Sylvia are not prosecutors but they are prosecuting Mrs. Obutu. Everybody seems friendly and interested in Sylvia's welfare, but all these strangers understand, with the precision of the English law, that Mrs. Obutu is guilty of being Sylvia's mother. For her, the court must seem full of enemies, speaking a foreign language. Does she understand that the magistrates want to hear her side of the story? Do they also have adolescent children? Does she think that at home, in Ghana, her husband would be the person in court, and that he would know how to respond to strange questions? We do not know, and we will never know. Since she is not accused of any wrong doing, she doesn't have legal defense. Feelings do not fit a 6″ x 12″ legal sheet.

She is alone in the witness box. All these people look alike. It's so difficult to read English faces—maybe her father would know. She would need to prepare food for the journey, and walking to court would take six to seven hours. Yes, her father would know. An elder, he is like the head magistrate. He also deals with family problems. He would tell these English that children owe respect to their parents. Sylvia must take care of the other two children while I take care of the baby. She is already fourteen years old and needs to be home. Her English friends are mixing her up. The other night she came in at 1 a.m. Of course she had to be beaten—children must obey their parents.

USHER (*giving her a written oath*): By what religion do you want to swear?
MRS. OBUTU: I am Christian.

The usher selects from a pile of books the Bible of the Church of England. Mrs. Obutu swears to tell the truth, nothing but the truth . . . what truth?

LAWYER: You heard the testimony of Mrs. Bennett saying that you beat your daughter with a stick.

MRS. OBUTU: I never beat my daughter with a stick. I want my daughter back. She needs to help me. My husband is in Ghana.

LAWYER: Did you beat her with your hands?

MRS. OBUTU: I have two other children at home; one is five, the other eight. She needs to help me with the children. I will not hit her again.

LAWYER: So you do admit that you have beaten her. Did you beat her with a stick?

MRS. OBUTU: I was born in Ghana. I need my daughter. She goes to the supermarket to buy the food. I will not hit her again.

LAWYER: You heard Mrs. Bennett saying that Sylvia said you hit her with a stick and once with a shoe.

MRS. OBUTU: Sylvia is having bad friends. She was caught by the police shoplifting. The police came to my home. I was ashamed; she meets bad people; I had to hit her.

LAWYER: So on this particular occasion, you did hit her. Did you lose your temper?

MRS. OBUTU: I was ashamed.

LAWYER: Do you hit your other children?

MRS. OBUTU: I never hit my children. I will not hit Sylvia again. I need my daughter.

LAWYER: Does your husband hit your children?

MRS. OBUTU: No, he never hit the children. I was frightened.

LAWYER: You were angry?

MRS. OBUTU: I was born in Ghana. Give me back my daughter.

HEAD MAGISTRATE: It's all right, Mrs. Obutu, you can go down and sit in your chair.

Mrs. Obutu goes back to her chair, near Sylvia, who has been holding the baby. She takes the baby in her lap and looks at the friendly face of the magistrate. Did she do well? Did the judge understand that she was ashamed when the social worker took Sylvia away? The face of the judge remains friendly. She must have done well. The three magistrates consult with each other and read two reports that Sylvia's lawyer has passed to the bench.

HEAD MAGISTRATE: Mrs. Obutu, here it says that Sylvia is doing very well in school.

MRS. OBUTU: But the police came to my house.

HEAD MAGISTRATE: Yes, I know, but the teacher says that Sylvia is a good girl, that she likes her. Mrs. Obutu, could you leave the room so that we can talk with Sylvia? (*Mrs. Obutu, alarmed, remains seated.*)

HEAD MAGISTRATE (*to usher*): Can you accompany Mrs. Obutu out? (*To Mrs. Obutu*) I will tell you later anything you need to know.

Mrs. Obutu leaves and Sylvia goes to the witness box. She reads the oath with difficulty.

LAWYER: Sylvia, where were you born and how old are you?

SYLVIA: I was born in London and I am fourteen and a half years old.

LAWYER: Can you tell the magistrate why you ran away the 12th of October?

SYLVIA: The police came to my home and asked my mother to come to the station. I was in the station because the police took me and my friend from Woolworths because we took two lipsticks without paying. My mother began to beat me in the street in front of my friend, and I ran away.

LAWYER: Did your mother beat you before?

SYLVIA: She beats me when she gets angry.

LAWYER: Did she beat you with a stick?

SYLVIA: She once beat me with a stick in the hand, the stick broke. I still have the scar (she indicates her left hand).

LAWYER: Where else does she beat you?

SYLVIA: Sometimes in the back.

LAWYER: Some other place?

Sylvia understands that she is not satisfying the lawyer's precise legal accounting and hurries her thinking processes.

SYLVIA: Once she beat me on the head (*her loyalty toward her mother makes her qualify her statement*), but that was a long time ago.

LAWYER: Where do you want to live?

SYLVIA: I don't know.

2ND LAWYER: Do you want to go back home with your mother?

SYLVIA: No, I don't want to go back home.

2ND LAWYER: What would you do if we sent you back home?
SYLVIA (*in a fast, rehearsed answer*): I will run away.

The judge indicates that Sylvia can step down, and the lawyer makes a summation indicating that it is clear that Section 2 is more precise in Paragraph F than in Paragraph E, but this can be remedied by Article D. Since everybody seems to understand the meaning of the code, Mrs. Obutu is called back to court. Meanwhile, the magistrates confer among themselves and seem to reach an agreement.

HEAD MAGISTRATE: Mrs. Obutu, we have come to the decision to put Sylvia in the care of the Borough of St. Vincent. We hope that you will visit your daughter, and she can go to your home to visit you and her siblings.

Mrs. Obutu, forgetting she is a foreigner playing in a game with foreign rules, jumps from her chair and stalks toward the bench; there, standing with her legs apart and her arms above her head, she roars: "I will not accept that. Sylvia is my daughter, you cannot take her away. I am from Ghana. My husband is from Ghana. I didn't die so you can't take her away from me. I didn't die; take me if you want, take the baby! Take all of us!"

For a brief moment, the court is in retreat. Who is this African queen mother challenging their own Queen's rule? She cannot say, "I will not accept that." This is against the rules. The clerk moves forward in his fast calypso rhythm, as if to protect the sanctity of the bench. The magistrates take a dignified retreat to the inner chambers, and Mrs. Obutu remains in the middle of the room, without an audience. She continues roaring, but it is clear even to her that her voice is dying against the walls of the court. Slowly, with her head low, she takes the baby and goes out, leaving Sylvia behind.

The magistrates return, looking upset. Not because Mrs. Obutu roared in pain; in their many years on the bench, pain has become a frequent witness in the chamber and they have learned how to deal with it. Justice provides them with an electronic scrambler to dissect pain into its logical components and to eliminate passion. No, they are upset because their sympathies are with Mrs. Obutu. They understood, because all of them are parents, that Mrs. Obutu is a Ghanian mother trying her best with her English daughter. Cultural gaps are familiar to them. But they were caught in their own legal structure. Nobody protected Mrs. Obutu from giving evidence against herself. Nobody defended her because she wasn't accused. Nobody represented Mrs. Obutu's other three children, who were losing Sylvia's affection, companionship, and care. Nobody represented Mr. Obutu. And certainly it didn't occur to anybody to have Mrs. Obutu and Sylvia talk to each other in the court to put in evidence for the magistrates the conflicting sets of loyalties, affection, care, frustration, and rage that characterized their relationship. Just as in all families. So, with a sense of doing an injustice, they cut off the left limb of the Obutu family and gave it "in care" to British social services.

Mrs. White

The court quickly settles back to business. But there seems to be some procedural holdup. The three magistrates confer again, heads close. The clerk hovers nearby, eager to help. Finally they reach some decision. The clerk straightens up. "Mrs. White?" she calls.

A woman enters quickly, followed by two little girls. The head magistrate smiles, acknowledging their presence. "Thank you, Mrs. White," he says in his friendly way. "You may be seated. Deborah, Grace. You have been here before." It is neither a question nor a statement, just part of the greeting ritual. "This case was brought last month," one of the lawyers reminds the judge. The judge nods. "Do we need the children?" The lawyer says no. "Off you go," the judge says cheerfully. He lifts his hands, palms up, in a gesture of dismissal. The children get up and leave with a social worker.

The lawyer reads drily from notes, summarizing the case. The mother was found drunk. Mr. Lewis from the House Association entered the apartment. The children seemed afraid, the police were called, the children removed to a "place of safety." Mrs. White sits straight and prim, as though she would like to believe they are talking about someone else. I remember now that I noticed the White family earlier in the waiting room. Mrs. White arrived alone. Each of the girls also came separately, accompanied by a social worker. The girls' social workers whispered to them, indicating that they should sit with their mother. Grace, who seems about eight, carried a satchel of books, coloring books, and a jigsaw puzzle. They sat next to their mother, three ladies in a row, all proper and prim. Grace tried to keep Deborah occupied, making sure she did not fidget. All three of them seemed tense, waiting.

Probably they all woke up very early this morning. Perhaps Grace woke up afraid . . . "I'll see Mommy today, in court. But Mommy will be angry. In the month I've been in the children's home, Mommy came to visit only twice. She was nice during the visits, but the other children say that Mrs. Cook is always watching, from the windows in her office, to make sure that mothers don't hit their children. Maybe Mommy was nice because she knew the staff were watching her. The people in the home are nice, especially Mrs. Cook. She sits with us while we eat. She has six children, and the youngest is eight, like me. And she grew up in Jamaica, like Mommy. But when Mommy drinks, she gets ugly. That night Mr. Lewis came, Mommy held me like a baby, and kissed me, and wanted to give me a baby bottle, then pat me on the back. I was afraid. I'm not a baby. Deborah is younger, and she's too big for a bottle. Mr. Lewis asked me if Mommy was hitting us, because I was crying, and Debbie was crying, and Mommy was laughing. I told him I was afraid, because when Mommy drinks, she doesn't know what she's doing. When Daddy lived with us she didn't drink, because he'd get mad if there was even one bottle of beer in the fridge. But he went away, and now she drinks, and gets ugly. And today we have to go to court, and the judge will say we can go home. Mommy will be nice in court, but then she'll be ugly. I told Mrs. Cook, but she said I have to go home, to help Mommy. I told her I do help her, but I'm afraid when she's ugly. She told me to tell the judge; maybe someone can help her with her drinking. I'll tell the judge. I hope Mommy doesn't get mad."

When Deborah opened her eyes, she immediately began studying the cloud shapes on the ceiling. In the month she had been at the Child Assessment Center, she had become familiar with those shapes. There was one like a whale. If she squinted, she could make it squirt water from the nose whales have on the back of their heads. She turned her head and looked at Sebille, who had crawled into bed with her. Sebille was much younger, of course: only four. Sebille has nightmares, and sometimes when she wakes up frightened, she comes to Debbie's bed. Debbie, at five and a half, doesn't have nightmares any more. It makes her feel good to be like an older sister.

Today Deborah would not go to school. She would dress in her best clothes, to go to court. Mommy and Grace would be there too. And today the judge would tell them they could go home. This is all Grace's fault! If she hadn't told the social workers that Mommy hits her when she drinks, they wouldn't have sent her to this place. *She* didn't tell the social worker anything! She'll tell Mommy that. And when the judge asks her, she'll tell him that she wants to be home with Mommy. She puts on the shiny new shoes that Mrs. Beck gave her, combs her hair, and washes her ears, so the judges will see that she can take care of herself. And if they ask her if she wants to go home, she'll say yes. She hopes the judges won't ask Grace, because when Grace gets angry she curses; and the judge will think they aren't good and keep her in this place.

Mrs. White dresses in her Sunday best bought three years ago, a brown tweed suit with a yellow blouse. It is discreet and gives a touch of middle-class businesswoman to her brown skin, something like a teacher or a nurse. She drinks a cup of black coffee to take away the smell of her last beer. She opens the door of the fridge and looks at the two six-packs in it; she likes her beer cool even in winter. But this is going to be the end of it. She is going to finish this beer and quit. It has been her ruin really. First her husband left her last year, after eleven years of marriage, and now social workers have taken away Deborah and Grace. It isn't worth it. This time she is going to do it, absolutely cold turkey; she will finish the six-packs and never touch a drop after that. She isn't a drunk! Here and there on social occasions she likes to drink, just to be happy and mix with people. It is true lately that, when she was down, she would sit at home and drink beer, but only when she felt really miserable. But it is her own home, and it isn't any-body's business. It was wrong for Mr. Lewis from the Council to come to her home and call the police. She wasn't doing anything wrong. Her house is well-kept, she always pays her rent on time, mops and shines her section of the hall and the stairs. He didn't have any right to enter her house and question the children. He would not have allowed *her* to ask his children about *his* life! And now Deborah and Grace have been away a month, and in differ-ent homes, they who are so close—like twins, if it weren't for the difference in age. She wonders how Deborah is doing. Grace can manage, she is very strong-willed, but Deborah has nightmares and cries at night.

But today is the day in court, and by this afternoon the girls will be back with her. The social worker told her that the emer-gency order was only good for twenty-eight days. Mrs. White opens the fridge and drinks a bottle of beer to calm her nerves. She'll finish the other eleven bottles, and that will be the end of it.

The lawyer has reached the end of his summation now. It states that counsel has not had time to make a complete investigation. An interim court order is requested—an extra month, to give counsel time to investigate. Mrs. White stiffens in silent protest, but no one is looking at her. The magistrates are asking the law-yer for the children if she has any objection. The lawyer says there is no objection. The judge asks Mrs. White courteously if it will be convenient for her to meet again in one month. She stands, smiles, and leaves the court, still smiling. The whole procedure has lasted eight minutes. The White family will remain in limbo, for an-other month.

Elizabeth Roberts

The clerk calls the next case. My neighbor hastily reaches into his briefcase and pulls out a sheet of paper. I glance in his direction; he shrugs and hands me the brief. It is a "C.Y.P. 7" bearing two impressive crowns, one with the legend "Honi soit qui mal y pense." All the power of the Crown, and even of God, is brought to bear on:

Joan and Jeffrey Roberts (the relevant infants)
Elizabeth Roberts (parent)

The "relevant infants" are to be brought before the Roxborough Juvenile Court under Section 1, Children and Young Persons Act, 1969, "since it is alleged that their proper development is being avoidably prevented or neglected or their health is being avoidably impaired or neglected or they are being ill treated. It is further alleged that the relevant infants are in need of care or control which they are unlikely to receive unless the Court makes an order under S [1]." The form is of course properly signed. There is a postscript after the signature: "If you wish to be legally represented you may apply to the Chief Clerk, Inner London Juvenile Courts, for particulars of legal aid which may be granted by the court." The postscript is a reminder that this is London, in the 1980s, a civilized city in a democratic society, where the rights not only of the "relevant infants" but also of their accused mother shall be upheld.

Elizabeth is ushered through the door. "She's only a child," I think, startled. But when this child was fifteen she engaged in the creation of another. Without much thought—in fact, to her mild surprise—she became pregnant. Her pregnancy was confirmed when the fetus was six months old. She reacted to the news the way she had learned to react to all the events of her life—with apathy. The father of the child-to-be was a youngster her age, with whom she'd had a short affair. She considered telling him about the child and then decided not to. This was going to be her baby. For Elizabeth, who didn't have too many possessions in her life, it was a chance to own something. A few months later she owned a baby, a new page in her large dossier in the welfare office, and a new social worker.

Elizabeth's own mother, an orphan who started her maternal career around the same age, was not pleased at becoming a grandmother at the age of thirty. She had two other children, was unmarried, and worked in a bakery. She had taken care of her two other daughters most of her life, but Elizabeth, the product of her early adolescence, had spent most of her life "in care." Sometimes "in care" seems like one of those euphemisms the English use—like "industrial action"—that mean the opposite. When Elizabeth was six months old she went to St. George's Children's

Home. She remembers the place very well. It was her home on and off until she was eight. She loved the staff, and they loved her. The only problem was that she always lost them. Sometimes that happened when she was taken home, whenever her mother felt she could cope with her. Sometimes it happened when staff members left the institution. Elizabeth learned to protect herself; if she didn't want to be hurt, she'd better not love anybody. This was difficult when she was young, but she kept trying. She kept re-learning and trying again. She tried again when she was sent to another institution at the age of nine, and at eleven when she was sent to the Jeffrey School for Children, and still later in another institution whose name she can't remember. She made a mistake in loving one set of foster parents, who loved her. They split up, and she moved to another institution. Sometimes she tries to re-member the names of some of these places, and how long she was there, but the days and events keep jumping around until it all blurs into one life interrupted by dozens of people who were sup-posed to be important to her.

One memory emerges. When she was fourteen years old, she was sent to a school for "maladjusted girls." She can still see it. Her mother and her social worker are talking with a tall man. There are other people around, and she knows they are talking about her, though she can't hear what they are saying. After two months at the school, Elizabeth learns what it is. She is hurt by the injustice. She is not maladjusted. Maladjusted girls behave badly. They don't know how to talk to people. It's not fair! But for the most part Elizabeth has protected herself by not reacting very much. She was never good at school, so her reading is la-borious, but she has learned other things that have served her well in her short life. One of them has to do with power, or lack of it. She knows that things happen to her because other people want them to happen. So she accepts life pretty much as it is imposed on her. That is how she accepted the arrival of Jeffrey, some two years after the birth of Joan. With Jeffrey, she acquired a Coun-cil flat and still another social worker, Alan, a nice-looking, con-cerned, twenty-four-year-old man. Alan had not yet accepted the way life plays Russian roulette with the powerless. He knew who held the gun, and he was determined to lend Elizabeth some of his anger as a tool against hopelessness and despair.

Elizabeth has never understood what Alan means. She isn't

hopeless, just accepting. There are times when she can't accept any more, when her cup is really full, when she can't cope with Joan and the baby and is afraid of venting her nervousness on them. At such times, Elizabeth escapes. She goes to her room, closes the door, takes a razor blade, and begins to cut her wrist. She starts with scratches, just surface stuff, and then goes for deeper cuts. This is why she prefers blunt blades. The sharp ones cut so easily you don't really feel it, and Elizabeth wants to feel what she is doing. The psychiatrist says that Elizabeth is depressed. Alan is afraid she will kill herself one of these days. Elizabeth doesn't agree. Cutting herself is not a matter of death but of life. When Elizabeth takes her blunt razor blades and begins to cut slowly, when she feels the pain and sees the scratches and the blood, she is then convinced that she has the power to make things happen. She has told Alan so many times, but he is still angry at her. He takes her to the hospital and then calls to check that she keeps her appointment to have the dressings changed.

Last time, Alan made Elizabeth promise she wouldn't cut herself again. She promised. That's another thing Elizabeth has learned to do—but how can a puppet keep her word when she doesn't know how the strings are controlled? Last week she did it again, and this time Alan is really mad. That's why they are in court. Alan is in the witness box.

ALAN: Last Monday, the 10th of November, Elizabeth called me at my home at 11 p.m. and told me she'd cut her wrists again. I rushed to her flat and found her sitting in the living room, holding Jeff in her lap, with blood all over her. For a moment, I thought she had cut the baby, but it was all her blood. I took the children to a neighbor and then took Elizabeth to the emergency room. She stayed the night and was discharged the next day. I am now concerned for the safety of the children, mostly Jeff. As I stated in the report, I recommend that he be put in care, and that Elizabeth and Joan go to a day hospital.

MAGISTRATE: Where would you put Jeff? He isn't even two.

ALAN: He has been with a foster family in Islington for four weeks. I recommend he remain there.

MAGISTRATE: Isn't that too far from the mother?

ALAN: It's one hour by car, and about an hour and a half by public transportation. Besides, Jeff would be brought to the day hospital every week for play therapy.

The magistrate looks at Elizabeth, shrunken in her chair, her eyes vacant, staring into a future without her baby.

MAGISTRATE (*friendly*): Elizabeth, do you want to say something?
ELIZABETH: No.

This is another one of the valuable lessons Elizabeth has learned—don't prolong events with hope. Events are bitter, so keep them short. She knows the decision has already been made. The magistrates retire to chambers. When they return they agree with Alan and with Jeff's lawyer, and start the third generation of the Roberts family "in care."

There are no other cases; the court closes around 1 p.m. I sit puzzled. The dramas I have witnessed just don't make sense. The human suffering is immeasurable. The costs of the procedure and the future decisions will be enormous. The magistrates are decent people. The social workers are committed, engaged professionals. The lawyers truly believe that they act for "the best interests of the child." How does all this good will result in such a carnage of dismemberment?

It seems that society's legal response to violence in the family is always one of control. Mrs. Obutu's beating of her adolescent daughter, Mrs. White's tipsy slapping, and Elizabeth's depression get the same legal response. Since violence is all of a piece, so is the reaction: restrain the victimizer and remove the victim to safety. But in family situations this response punishes both the victimizer and the victim.

If we understood violence better, could we respond more effectively? Emanuel Marx, an Israeli sociologist who has studied violent behavior in an immigrant village, creates a distinction that may be useful in describing families and might serve courts as well. He observes that one pattern is characterized by purposeful, controlled violence; it involves the use of threat and the escalation of violence to achieve a goal. This pattern he calls *coercive violence*. In families, the most common example would be that of parents beating their children as part of their socialization efforts, but in many social and political negotiations as well, the threat and utilization of force become an important part of the geography of the transaction.

There is another type of violence seen more frequently in families who come in contact with the law and the mental-health profession: violence in which the victimizer perceives himself or herself as a victim. In this second type, *pleading violence* ("appealing violence" in Marx's terminology), "the violent person demonstrates that society has treated him unfairly, for instance by making demands on him which are incompatible with the resources placed at his disposal." In families characterized by child abuse or spouse beating, perpetrators of the violent act often experience themselves as helpless responders to the other person's baiting. In these circumstances, the "helpless victimizer" pleads for an increased understanding of his or her impossible plight. Regardless of our emotional response to such a distortion of facts, it is obvious that punitive control of this kind of violent person will increase the subjective experience as a victim and will maximize the chance of further violence.

Looking back at the families I saw in court, it is clear that only Mrs. Obutu exercised coercive violence. She wanted her daughter to mend her ways and used force as a reminder. In none of the other three cases was there "purpose" to the violent act. This seems to me to be true of most cases of violence in families. Consider, for instance, a family with a violent adult son who terrorized the family. The father described himself to me this way:

> I am a very peaceful man. All my life people I deal with have been able to reason with me. But when I'm at home and I say something perfectly sensible or I suggest something that is absolutely right and my wife rejects it, I become violent (*he shakes his fist at his wife*) because she makes me meaningless and I can't accept that.

The son, in turn, described himself this way:

> I have never been violent outside my home. But sometimes my father *pushes me* into violence. The other day I was making a cup of tea, and he switched off the stove. I grabbed him and pushed his head out the fourth-floor window. He wanted to tell me that he is number one. I know I'm less than zero. He doesn't have to tell me.

Both father and son see themselves as victims, and their violence is not directed toward the implementation of a goal. It is a plea for the understanding of their hopeless situation in life.

In another situation, a mother reviewing her history as a child abuser described her relationship with her infant in this way:

MOTHER: I would dread her coming back from the daycare center.

MINUCHIN: What did you feel?

MOTHER: I was dreading her rejecting me . . . the food I gave her, her saying no to me. That would spark my violence.

M: What was the feeling?

MOTHER: "How dare you say no to me? No to something I give you?" And because she was little, I became powerful and she became even smaller. It was as if I could squeeze her and throw her in the trash.

M: What prompted the feeling of wanting to smash her?

MOTHER: I wanted to feel my physical power. I got pleasure in feeling control. At times she didn't have to say a word. If I wanted to feel powerful, I would snap at her. She would do everything at my beck and call. "Do this," and she did it. "Yes, Mommy. Okay, Mommy." And that was pleasure.

If the inquiry were stopped at this point, we would locate the violence in the mother and see its implementation as pleasurable. Our response to that focus would have to be the control of the mother and removal of the child. But, if we broaden our perspective, a more complex pattern appears.

MOTHER: If she rejected my food, I sat literally fuming. How dare she? I had invested time. She was saying no to me, not just the food. I would lose control and ram the food down her throat till she choked.

M: Did she do something to make you stop? From where did the signal come that made you stop?

MOTHER: It came from within myself. I said, "Continue like that, and you'll kill her. Stop now." But I didn't want to. I wanted her to submit. She was going to eat and I was going to make her do that.

Here we see a transactional pattern between mother and daughter, a power operation between a year-and-a-half-old child and a thirty-year-old mother. In a strange alchemy, the wish to give love was transformed into a helpless, destructive act; and the cycle of provocation and violence escalated.

M: What did your husband do to control or provoke your rage?

MOTHER: The rage didn't come when he was there because I knew he wouldn't take it. He always sided with her. I hated him for siding with her and not seeing that she'd asked for that food, she'd specifically asked for it, and now she was telling me no. She was rejecting me, and he was on her side!

M: What did you do with your rage toward your husband?

MOTHER: I only attacked him once. I threw a plate at him.

HUSBAND: Once I wasn't in the mood to listen to her. I slapped her in the face and went out. I heard the plate hit the door.

MOTHER: I had been hit so much in my life as a child. Now I'm an adult, and they're still doing it to me.

M (to husband): What was your feeling toward her when she was violent?

HUSBAND: When she was violent with the child, I was violent with her.

MOTHER: When he was angry, he yelled at me. He sounded very very vicious and though he never actually laid a hand on me, I felt that at any moment he was going to smash me. I screamed and shouted at him, and didn't hear what he said. My feeling was that this gorilla is going to pull me to pieces. I was so afraid. I would plot how I could get a knife in the middle of the night and murder him.

M: When you were violent with your daughter, were you afraid that your husband would attack you?

MOTHER: I got to feeling as if I was crawling on the floor just like the baby. If he would say go get me a cup, I would dash off and get it for him. In my eyes, I was just doing to my daughter what he was doing to me.

Now the picture is more complex. The violence of the mother mirrors her situation with her husband. Helpless, afraid of his violence, she redresses the balance in acts of violence toward her daughter. Is she attacking her husband by attacking his ally? Or is the daughter the healer, allowing her to gain competence? Whichever way you interpret it, you cannot see this behavior as instrumental violence. There is no controlling goal to this violence. But let's look further.

MOTHER: I was a disappointment to my mother because I had a girl. I let down my family and my husband's family; they all wanted a boy. My mother wanted nothing to do with the baby. She was an unmarried mother herself. She went to her parents and was rejected. Now I was coming to her (this was before we got married), and she could only see herself again.

Now we can see a context that is even wider than the nuclear family: the mother's position as a woman in a culture where a woman has lower status, and her position within her family of origin and her husband's. The legal system responded to this mother as it did to Mrs. Obutu and the other women in the London court. It used the only intervention available, and the baby was "removed to a place of safety." Fortunately in this case, intensive multiple therapeutic input (a therapeutic nursery, family therapy, and individual therapy for the mother) was able to change the patterns in the family, which is functioning successfully today.

For the most part, society acts as if all family violence is instrumental, and the response therefore is to increase control. But it is clear to us as family therapists that most cases of family violence are the products of generations of powerlessness. When we try to intervene by controlling the parents or with concern for the child alone, we can only produce a continuation of the pattern.

READER: Ideologues scare me. I swear some of you would sell your mothers just to prove a point about filial love.
AUTHOR: Why are you suddenly calling me names?
READER: Because you select reality to conform to your own point of view. Systemic solutions to family violence are acceptable only if you deny its destructiveness.
AUTHOR: I can't deny it. I've seen it too many times.
READER: With children?

AUTHOR: Yes, and I agree with you. The statistics on child abuse are bad enough. When you actually see a child with broken bones, or third-degree burns, or hungry, or just looking at you with those vacant eyes that tell you—

READER: Then I'm intrigued. If you still insist on a systemic approach even when children are being abused, how can you possibly object to being called an ideologue?

AUTHOR: I would prefer to be called a person with a way of looking at the world of violence. I've had to deal with family violence, and my first response in a case of child abuse or incest has always been to protect the child. I often recommend family dismemberment for that reason. But unlike the judicial system, I then continue to look at what happens. And what I've seen following this solution is often more violence. What can you do when you close your eyes and, when you open them, the reality of violence is still waiting?

READER: I think that this is only part of the reality—that there is more.

AUTHOR: I get furious. I despair. The power of institutions to maintain themselves after it has become clear that they are destructive . . .

READER: Hold on there. What do you expect me to do with this anger?

AUTHOR: I want you to help me scream. Maybe together we could yell a little louder.

Child Murder

Maria Colwell

(10) Maria Colwell was born on the 25th March 1965, so that when she died at the hands of her stepfather, William Kepple, on the night of the 6th/7th January 1973 she was eleven weeks short of her eighth birthday.

This is the beginning of the Narrative of the *Report of the Committee of Inquiry into the Care and Supervision Provided in Relation to Maria Colwell*, printed by Her Majesty's Stationery Office in London in 1974. The single sentence encompasses Maria Colwell's entire life. But the report on her death is 120 closely printed pages, with carefully numbered paragraphs. What did a child dead at seven do to rate such a heavy epitaph?

At the age of six Maria was a polite, well-dressed little girl, perhaps slightly spoiled. But in October 1971 she was removed from the care of her foster parents and "returned" to her natural mother, Mrs. Kepple. Over the next year at least seventy-five people, including an assortment of child-welfare professionals, were involved in her case. Thus when her battered, starved body was pronounced dead on January 7, 1973, her death called the entire structure of the British child-welfare system into question.

(147) The post mortem carried out by Professor Cameron on 11 January showed that she was severely bruised all over the body and head and had sustained severe internal injuries to the stomach. There was a healing fracture of one rib. The bruising, which was described by Professor Cameron as the worst he had ever seen, was of variable age . . . but the majority dated from within 48 hours. The majority of the

injuries he described as the result of extreme violence. The stomach was empty and the body weighed 36 lbs, whereas . . . she should for her age and height have weighed anything between 46 and 50 lbs.

How could a child who was officially under the eye of the Brighton Social Services Department, the East Sussex Social Services Department, and the National Society for the Prevention of Cruelty to Children have been so maltreated over a period of months? A Committee of Inquiry was appointed to gather the answers to that question. As Joseph Goldstein, Anna Freud, and Albert Solnit later observed:

> The inquiry into her death was held in public in Brighton, Sussex. It lasted 41 days during which 70 witnesses were heard. While it caused considerable upset to the authorities and workers concerned, lessons learned from the inquiry triggered moves toward administrative changes and reformation of official and personal attitudes. According to one British social worker, practices in the Social Services can be divided into two eras: *before* and *after* Maria Colwell.

Unfortunately, the focus of the inquiry, and of the subsequent reforms, was the existing system and how to improve it.

I have chosen this case to discuss because it can also be used to demonstrate a different field of observation—how tunnel vision hampered both the recognition of Maria's danger and the possibility of intervention, ultimately resulting in her death. During her short life Maria sent many messages out that she was endangered and needed allies. These messages were heard by at least a hundred people: relatives, neighbors, and health professionals. She did not live in a world deaf to children crying. But the values of the social and legal systems scrambled her messages so badly that they could not be properly decoded. Looking at the Maria Colwell case from the point of view of a family therapist, I see a group of good people, including dedicated servants of social and legal services, who couldn't respond to Maria because they thought in fragmented ways. Their cognitive models imposed a kind of acoustical screen so that Maria's cries were absorbed and blunted. If I am right, then the reforms introduced to improve those legal and social service systems will only help to retain incorrect points of view. It is tragic that Maria's death and its consequences may prove prejudicial to other children and their families.

Maria was the fifth child of her mother's first marriage. Her father left her mother within weeks of her birth; he died a few weeks later. In December 1965 the court committed the four older children to the care of the East Sussex County Council. But Mrs. Colwell took the infant Maria to her sister-in-law, Mrs. Cooper. Eventually the Coopers were made Maria's foster parents, and she lived with them for the next six years, visited only irregularly by her biological mother.

As frequently happens in situations of prolonged foster care, a strong relationship developed between Maria and her foster parents, her aunt and uncle. It became much more significant than the tenuous contacts with her natural mother. As is also common in situations of this type, a triangular structure evolved, with Maria's mother and the Coopers competing for the rights of decision making in Maria's life. Maria was in the middle, caught between her love, affection, and belonging to the Coopers and her knowledge (maintained by the Coopers, the Council, and Mrs. Colwell) that she legally belonged to her mother.

In 1966 Maria's mother began to live with William Kepple, with whom she had three children, born in November 1967, December 1968, and November 1969. Maria's social context, therefore, became rather complex: she had four siblings, three half siblings, the Coopers and their children, Mrs. Tester (her maternal grandmother in whose care her older brother lived), the foster homes where the rest of her siblings lived, Mr. Kepple (her mother's paramour and later husband), and the East Sussex Council with its representatives in social services. A number of other agencies were to enter into Maria's life, and their intervention also affected the total organism of which Maria was a part.

In 1969, having established a relationship with Mr. Kepple that Social Services evaluated as "stable," Mrs. Colwell consulted a solicitor about applying for a revocation of the order assigning Maria to the care of the Coopers. It seemed clear to Social Services that Maria's emotional family was the Coopers, who wanted to adopt her. But the application of a natural mother who now had a home to offer her child was very likely to succeed. Social Services began to plan Maria's return to the Kepples.

It is interesting to trace the thinking behind Maria's return. Legally the situation was clear. Maria "belonged" to her natural mother. The Coopers, as mere foster parents, had no legal rights in this situation. They were not to be consulted or even officially informed about the disposition of Maria's case. To Social Services, these were simply the facts of the matter.

(35) The Coopers would of course be greatly distressed to lose Maria, but the present state of the law being what it is with foster parents in such a position having no rights, except perhaps in rare cases that of making the child a ward of court and allowing the High Court to decide what is best in the interests of the child, it was clearly impossible for the social workers to consider the Coopers' feelings in any decision they came to.

A case discussion reviewing the circumstances surrounding Maria and the prospects for her future concluded:

(36) It would seem that whatever the decision was taken concerning Maria it would involve stress and trauma for her at some time. On balance it was felt that future plans should be directed towards her eventual return to her mother ... It should be easier for her to build relationships with the Kepple family and to take her place within [it] at a younger age, particularly considering the good emotional grounding she has received from the Coopers.

In other words, Maria was now to be "transplanted"—Social Services' word—like a tree. Maria had been planted in good earth and carefully tended. Thus at the ripe age of six, she should be able to maintain that "good emotional grounding." But the metaphor ends here. Any gardener knows enough to keep a ball of earth around the roots of a plant while transplanting. But there was to be no attempt to carry earth from the Coopers to the Kepples. Maria, the Coopers, and the Kepples would all have to survive this transplant individually, mustering their individual strengths. There was to be no intervention to help the Kepples and Maria grow together. And for the Coopers, there would simply remain an empty hole:

(36) Whatever action is taken one or other of these people [the Coopers and Mrs. Kepple] will be hurt but it was felt help could be given with this and Maria's interests must be considered as of paramount importance.

This statement is dressed as objective truth. But it is actually a statement of faith. Look at what it says about:

(1) a style of bureaucratic inertia;
(2) self-justification and deception (if such "help" was ever actually planned, it disappeared under the pressures of sixty case workloads);
(3) socioeconomic blinders;
(4) professional jargon and mythmaking;
(5) a value system;
(6) a model of thinking about human processes.

What the law in its majesty was actually doing here is similar to dismembering a starfish or a flatworm, with the hope that the torn segments will grow. This can work well only with those animals. To Social Services' way of thinking, they were safeguarding "the best interests of the child." But conceptualizations and procedures based on a legal system designed to judge the claims of adversaries overrode human concerns that might have mitigated the pain of the situation, and perhaps saved Maria's life.

Any first-grader would recognize that the Kepples were a completely new factor in Maria's life. She was going to a new father, three new siblings, and a mother she had barely seen for six years. But legally this was a "return"—to Maria's natural environment and to the ownership of her natural mother. This was the first of a fatal series of moves made considering the child in isolation from her context, which is like playing chess with only one piece.

Move One: Maria's Return to the Kepples

During the summer of 1971 Social Services arranged several visits to help Maria get to know "her family." These were of questionable success—Maria ran away several times, threw screaming and hitting fits, and did everything in the power of a child of six to resist the visits, though the social worker noted that she seemed to enjoy herself once she was actually with her mother and stepsisters.

Mrs. Kepple slapped Maria "to make her understand it was wrong to run away." "I wish I lived on a farm in the country," Maria said. "No one would be able to find me there" (para. 53).

We are told very little about the Coopers' reaction to the imminent loss of Maria, though it is mentioned that Mrs. Cooper was "distressed." From a broader perspective, it seems clear that the Coopers/Maria system was having a bad time. Perhaps the Kepples were as well. When a family changes shape because of addition or removal of a member, the blueprints that regulate the transactions of the total organism change. This is a period of crisis, since the individual members find the familiar ways of working ineffective and there is no new way yet. Whether the result will be a more complex and harmonious pattern or a family still caught in old, stressful patterns depends on the way the family resources are mobilized. Transitional periods are points of new possibilities or of pain. For Maria, the Coopers, and the Kepples, only pain resulted.

> (54) By September the pattern was becoming well established. Regular visits were planned . . . and Maria's resistance was becoming more strenuous, resulting in major scenes on nearly every occasion. Two visits had to be cancelled because she had worked herself into such a state of kicking and screaming that [Maria's social worker] realised it was impossible to insist . . . On the other hand, it seemed that once arrived at the Kepples Maria tended to calm down and to enjoy the company of her siblings as well as continuing to forge an improved relationship with her mother.

> (56) On the 27th September after Maria had spent a weekend at the Kepples she returned with bruising in the form of distinct finger marks on her thigh and she told the Coopers that "the man who lived with Pauline [Mrs. Kepple] had done it."

But Mrs. Kepple was making it clear that she was not prepared to hold off making her application to the court for custody of Maria. Faced with Maria's imminent assignment to her mother's custody, Social Services decided that Maria's distress was

> (59) due to her fear of losing the Coopers rather than any fear or dislike of the Kepple household . . . in any event it was within expected and well recognised limits in such circumstances.

Here, in a nutshell, is the problem of the child-in-isolation model. It imposes an either/or dualism that doesn't encompass the complexity of human processes. In the attempt to achieve clarity, it polarizes. As a corollary of this model Social Services could not intervene in the social system of the Kepples and

Maria. It could only transplant the individual and then stand by, functioning mostly as observer and recorder of events. Unable to facilitate the growth of human systems, it functioned mostly as an arm of the court, amassing a record that ultimately filled some sixty-six pages of notes on ineffective attempts to protect Maria by surveillance of the Kepples. Losing its own language of support and humanitarianism, Social Services became part of a legal system whose code words are guilt, blame, and surveillance.

(64) Mrs. Kepple's application was to be heard on the 17th November and on the 22nd October Maria went back to Mrs. Kepple on trial. It is fair to record that two weeks before, [the social worker] on a visit to the Kepples was impressed with the very real efforts to improve the home which had been made recently and also with Mrs. Kepple's efforts at improving her own appearance. She thought the family was on a steady upward trend and the Kepple children were developing normally. On Friday the 22nd . . . Mr. Cooper . . . took [Maria] to the Hove Social Services Office whence Miss Coulthard . . . took her to the Kepples. She had screamed and clung to Mr. Cooper at the office and was apprehensive about going with her mother who was present. She was given an assurance by Mrs. Kepple in Miss Coulthard's presence that she would be returning to the Coopers at the weekend . . . She then went quietly and on that false note her new life began. She was never to see the Coopers again.

Move Two: Surveillance

The Kepple family had now been enlarged by one daughter. Within a few months, a number of new people began to join this larger organism.

(82) On Easter Monday, the 3 April, Mrs. Rutson, who lived next door to the Kepples, heard Mrs. Kepple shouting at Maria and calling her a "dirty little bitch" because she had dirtied herself, and this was followed by the repeated sounds of slapping.

(84) On Wednesday the 12 April . . . Mrs. Rutson looked up at the bedroom of number 119 . . . and saw Maria looking out of the side of the curtain. Her face was "terribly blackened and she had a terribly bloodshot eye—one eye was just a pool of blood . . ."

The next day Mrs. Rutson phoned the National Society for the

Prevention of Cruelty to Children, who sent an inspector. It was to be the first of complaints brought by over a dozen people, involving six separate agencies, during Maria's remaining eight months of life.

Mrs. Rutson informed the Kepples that she had reported them to the NSPCC. Mr. Kepple attacked Mrs. Rutson's father in the street. The police were called, and neighbors gave information on the Kepples to the investigating constable. Another neighbor called Social Services to complain that Maria was being beaten and locked in the house.

> (103) On or about the 24 April a deputation of the Kepples' neighbours complained to Mr. Smith of Brighton Housing Department under whose aegis came the administration of the Whitehawk estate. The complaints were of ill-treatment of Maria and that the Kepple children were encouraged to defecate out of doors.

Now we begin to see more of the ecology of this case. The neighbors are concerned adults. Outraged by Mr. Kepple's treatment of the children, particularly Maria, they resolve to defend them. The process, of course, results in various threats to the family. The Kepples live in Council housing; a complaint to the housing department threatens their shelter, which is bureaucratically connected to their only current source of income—Mrs. Kepple's dole and Mr. Kepple's disability payments. Even more fundamentally, Mrs. Kepple has already lost four children to the intervention of Social Services. Are the three she has been allowed to keep now threatened by these complaints and increased surveillance? Maria has many allies, up to and including the Crown itself. From the Kepples' point of view, Maria is endangering the well-being of the entire family.

The school enters the fray in February. Maria's teacher calls the social worker, voicing her concern that Maria is being used to run errands "at unsuitable times and to an extent entirely beyond her physical capacity." The Kepples are visited by representatives of the educational welfare office and a health officer. The neighbors' concern also builds. The local shopkeeper sends a message to Mrs. Kepple that she will no longer sell coal to Maria unless Maria is provided with some sort of conveyance for the heavy bag.

In November the Kepples go out for a beer, leaving the children alone in the house. A neighbor calls the police, who search the local public houses and then wait in the house until the Kepples finally return at 11 p.m. The parents are severely warned and later visited by a policewoman, who repeats the warning. Three days later the police again call, to make sure the warning has been heeded.

Move Three: The Paranoid System

The Kepple family were in a state of siege. And it seems highly probable that this closing circle of Maria's well-wishers intensified her danger. The Kepples may have felt themselves in a Kafkesque world full of accusers, frequently anonymous, complaining to vaguely defined but highly powerful authorities. In this kind of context, people often find it necessary to look for a target they can effectively attack. Accusers and authorities lie in shadow, but there is one person who is not only clearly responsible for their plight but also accessible: Maria.

(118) On the 7 November a deputation of neighbors waited upon Mr. Smith the area housing officer who had already received complaints in April about the Kepples. On this occasion they complained of drunkenness and nuisance by Mr. Kepple and of the children being left alone and they wanted the Kepples moved. On the 8 November Mr. Smith's assistant Mr. Topley visited the Rutson's house . . . and received a petition signed by various neighbours with the same objective. It listed a series of complaints about the Kepples including Mr. Kepple's drinking habit and the practice of his children of defecating out of doors . . . Mr. Kepple took the view it was nobody's business but his own. He agreed he drank too much on occasions and used the expression "free-range" with regard to his children's personal habits, which was his way of bringing them up . . . he clearly emphasized . . . a dislike of authority and a disregard for certain basic social standards.

(122) On the thirteenth of November Maria was late for school again and gave as the reason that she had to go shop for coal, bread and potatoes and [the educational welfare officer] visited that day but received no reply . . . Mrs. Turner, the teacher, had naturally been greatly shocked at the thought of a child of Maria's age and size hauling a 28 lb bag of coal up a steep hill, and her fears were in-

THE PARANOID SYSTEM

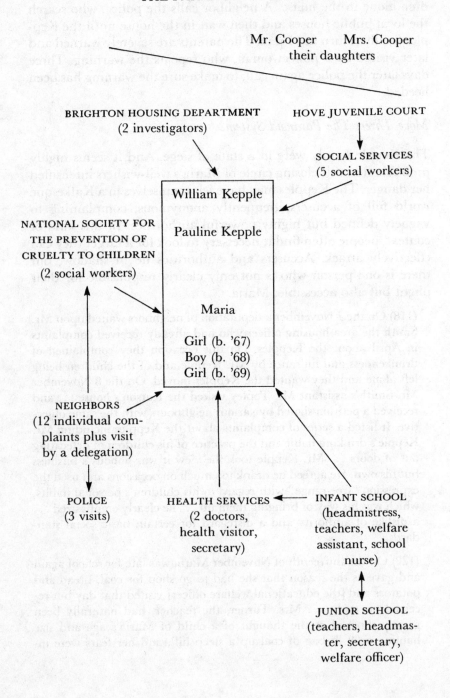

Mr. Cooper   Mrs. Cooper
their daughters

BRIGHTON HOUSING DEPARTMENT
(2 investigators)

HOVE JUVENILE COURT

SOCIAL SERVICES
(5 social workers)

William Kepple

Pauline Kepple

NATIONAL SOCIETY FOR
THE PREVENTION OF
CRUELTY TO CHILDREN
(2 social workers)

Maria

Girl (b. '67)
Boy (b. '68)
Girl (b. '69)

NEIGHBORS
(12 individual com-
plaints plus visit
by a delegation)

POLICE
(3 visits)

HEALTH SERVICES
(2 doctors,
health visitor,
secretary)

INFANT SCHOOL
(headmistress,
teachers, welfare
assistant, school
nurse)

JUNIOR SCHOOL
(teachers, headmas-
ter, secretary,
welfare officer)

creased a day or two later when Maria came up to her and said "Mommy says I have to tell you I did not go to the shop for coal. But honestly I did, Mrs. Turner."

We see here that Maria is searching for support against her family among the people who are sympathetic to her. The vicious circle is becoming smaller and smaller.

Move Four: Maria's Death

The month of December increased the involvement of the community. Now at last the bureaucracy began to move, sparked by the concern of Maria's teacher. Mrs. Kepple also made up her mind that the situation was impossible and told Mr. Kepple that she was going to tell Social Services that he and Maria didn't get on.

(146) However, on 6 January, which was a Saturday, Mr. Kepple came in at 11:30 p.m. and the events which formed the basis of the indictment against Mr. Kepple then occurred.

The following morning the Kepples brought Maria's body to the hospital, where she was pronounced dead.

Move Five: Aftermath

William Kepple was convicted of manslaughter; he received an eight-year sentence. Pauline Kepple developed a relationship with another man. A year later she was back in court, trying to obtain custody of her youngest child, in care at the age of five months. By this time she had borne ten children, of whom nine were in care. Two years later she was again in court, trying to get custody of her current baby. If Mrs. Kepple, who is still young and clearly fertile, continues to have a baby every thirteen or fourteen months, the legal system will undoubtedly continue to play the tragic game of waiting for every child she bears and putting it in care.

Move Six: Post Mortem

It is difficult to read the case of Maria Colwell, even ten years later, without great anger. There were many times when Maria's call could have been answered. But if anger were the only effect, there would be no point in recounting the story. The issue is not whether Maria would have been saved if she had been assigned to a different group of social workers, if her social worker had had a smaller caseload, or if various agencies had been in better communication. What can we learn from Maria, the Coopers, and the Kepples?

The inquiry into Maria's death confined itself to procedural conclusions. The committee investigated the way in which care and supervision had or had not been provided and the coordination of services. The report's concerns were communication among agencies, the communication within and between schools, between schools and Social Services departments, between Social Services and the National Society for the Prevention of Cruelty to Children, the police, the housing department, and so on. It examined the ways social workers communicate with children and keep records, and ended with a number of suggestions directed toward improving the system by weighting procedures more toward the best interests of the child. Nowhere is it suggested that the best interests of the child could be served better by interventions directed toward the context on which she is dependent.

A person who tries to look at the larger context, therefore, finds it remarkable how much information is left out of the report. We have no data on the relationship between Mr. and Mrs. Kepple. There is little information on the relationships between Maria, her parents, her siblings, and the extended family. Whenever information is given about the Kepples or Maria, they are described only in terms of their inner dynamics, not in terms of the transactions between them.

For Mr. Kepple, we don't even have much individual information. We are told he was an Irishman, the possessor of several aliases, and a "Bevin boy." Although it is nowhere stated, we are clearly given to understand that he was a Catholic. The report presents him as scornful of authority. The minority report by one member of the committee suggests that he was confused by the state's involvement in what he regarded as a purely private matter—the rearing of children. Was his forcing the children to defecate outside one way of commenting on the situation? Is it possible that beating Maria was a kind of declaration of independence?

What about Mrs. Kepple? Did she and Mr. Kepple fight about Maria? Did she try to protect Maria? Or did they join forces against her, as much of the neighbors' testimony suggests? What happened to the Coopers after Maria left? Maria ran away several times to their daughter, who lived within reach. What was the effect on that family?

The distinction drawn by Emanuel Marx brings an added dimension to the case of Maria Colwell. The system responded as it always does, as if this were a case of coercive violence, to be controlled through surveillance, warning, and punishment. As a result, the Kepples may have seen themselves as victimized by Maria. Their attack on her may have been a distorted plea for an understanding of their position. In effect, beating Maria may have been an expression of outrage and fear: "See what is being done to us."

It is difficult to take a positive view and impossible to sympathize with the murderers of a child. But unless we begin to see cases like Maria's not from the point of view of fixing the blame, but from the point of view of possible solutions, we will still be doomed only to the repetition of ineffective interventions. In Maria's individual case, it seems that the insistence on returning Maria to her natural mother was the root cause of her death. But let us generalize and postulate that Maria's problem actually started when she was put in care with the Coopers. Perhaps better solutions lie in changing our concepts of foster care.

Whenever I think of foster care, I find myself thinking of my Aunt Sofia. When my mother grew severely depressed after the death of her mother, I'm told, though I don't remember it myself, that my infant sister and I were sent for some time to Aunt Sofia, to give my mother space to recover and quite probably to ensure that we were adequately cared for. During the economic crises of the thirties my mother farmed us out for a while, again to Aunt Sofia. We were instructed to eat well before returning to our routine of polenta and bread at home.

On neither occasion did my relatives or my mother call this foster care. They wouldn't have known the word. My aunt didn't think that my parents were doing a poor job or that she had to compensate for them; neither did my parents. In my family it was taken for granted that relatives functioned as a system of support. Our household was frequently augmented by cousins, who came from the city to spend the two or three summer months in the country. During my childhood, my parents brought one of my mother's distant relatives from Russia to live with us; she stayed for a number of years until she married, I think. Families were supposed to be available to members of the clan. They were supposed to help.

These incidents from my family have been repeated all over the world across the centuries. Nuclear families are rarely isolated units; they are aggregates of the larger, extended organism. The utilization of "substitute" families for children in need is a natural response taken by most communities and cultures. Thus, when the child welfare and mental health movements began to use foster families, they were replicating an experiment that society has conducted in natural forms through many cultures. Foster care, particularly the placement of orphans, was a positive alternative to institutionalizing needy children.

Unfortunately, what started as a progressive orientation has degenerated into a dumping ground. By its very nature a short-term solution, foster care is all too often the only solution for children in care until they reach the age of legal adulthood, by which time, like Elizabeth Roberts and her boyfriends, they may have become "cases" in their own right.

The idea, of course, is to save the child, who is removed from the natural family, putting distance between the child and the noxious family environment. The traumatic effect that the separation produces on the children is recognized, but only rarely are the secondary impacts of displacement from familiar habitats and circumstances given serious consideration. The effects that the separation produces on the total family are not part of the mental-health literature; they don't figure in the legal system's area of responsibility.

It doesn't have to be that way. Common as foster care is, historically it is a relatively new legal solution. Phillippe Aries, in *Centuries of Childhood*, points out that in Europe prior to the fifteenth century children were considered miniature adults. They had the same legal rights and responsibilities. During the sixteenth century children began to be thought of as innocents requiring separation and protection from the adult world, but childhood as a social issue appeared only in the nineteenth century. Only then did we see the official placement of children in "foster arrange-ments." While the ritual of the London magistrates' court seems oiled by centuries, it has actually been in operation for less than a decade. It is the model that came into existence after the cases of Maria Colwell and others produced exploratory committees directed to streamline and improve the British Social Services re-sponse to children at risk. This replaced an earlier model, which replaced another; different social organizations bring into being their own views of children, families, and society.

What is our own society's concept of responsibility? In 1970, 3.8 per 1000 children in the United States were placed in foster care. Many studies documented the harm being done—establishing the following facts.

(1) Little effort is made to avoid placement. Alan Gruber's study of foster care in Massachusetts reports that 93 percent of the natural families interviewed felt that no strategies to keep their children at home had been considered by agencies prior to place-ment. In many cases a specific crisis precipitated foster care; the families reported they had been unable to receive assistance until the crisis was upon them and placement was pending. Gruber also reported that 90 percent of the placements were due to parental difficulties rather than to disability or behavioral problems on the part of the child.

(2) Once the child leaves the natural family, little is done to re-turn him or her to the family.

(3) During placement, the contact between children and their natural parents is minimal.

(4) Once a child is placed in a foster home, the likelihood of re-turn to the natural family decreases in proportion to the length of time away. Yet there is little long-range planning. Gruber re-ported that in Massachusetts 83 percent of the children were never returned to their natural family even for a trial period.

What if we could open avenues that are less traumatic for the child and the family, produce more effective results, and in the end are less financially burdensome? The idea is simple enough if, instead of looking only at the family's destructive effects on the child, we also consider its capacity to grow and heal.

What if the families who accept children in care were organized to become foster families for *families?* The parents in the foster family would be trained to take total family organization into account and to work foremost to eliminate the need for placement or facilitate the return of the child to the family of origin. Foster families would learn, in other words, to look at children in context and, in effect, to copy the extended family model. Under this type of focus, foster families could become professional participants in the mental-health and child-welfare system of care. The principal achievement of this approach would be to shift emphasis from intervention and maintenance to prevention. Such a program might also facilitate an earlier return of children to their natural families. Only one major change is necessary: a shift in orientation away from "rescuing children" toward the concept of "helping families."

The established model of thinking sharply separates the child in placement from the natural family, even while both law and guidelines "uphold" the natural parents' rights so stringently that many otherwise adoptable children spend their childhood in one foster family after another.

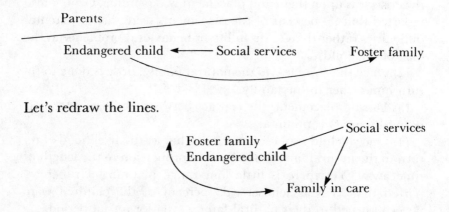

Let's redraw the lines.

With such a perspective, success would be measured not in survival, but in rehabilitation of the child in his family.

Suppose further that each family that took two to four children and their families in care were given clinical supervision. Two to four fostering families could organize themselves into a kin network connected to a child-guidance clinic or other sponsoring agency, forming a true institution without walls.

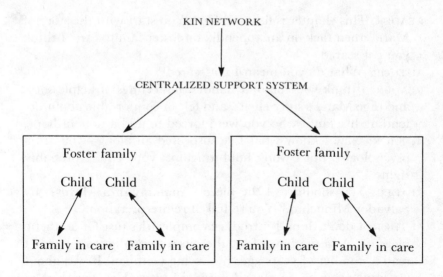

The way an institution like this would work would vary depending on the orientation of the central agency and the level of training of the foster families. But the model itself imposes certain directions.

(1) The foster family would have experiential information on the behavior of the child they foster and knowledge about the family culture that supports this behavior.

(2) Successful working with a child and her family would require the development of a better adjustment of the child in a growth-encouraging family context.

(3) Success of the involvement would be measured in successful rehabilitation of the child in his family.

(4) The extended family module would become a network for family support and a laboratory for social planning and experimentation.

Such a model would not require more funding and manpower than are poured into the current system. But I doubt that foster-care services will change. The established models of thinking and the established manpower that supports them will prevail in spite of the deaths of the Marias of this world and the cries of thousands of children and parents. It is a frightening comment on the power of the familiar.

READER: This chapter is fish and fowl. You start with the story of Maria, then tack on an appendix on foster-family care. I think you got scared.

AUTHOR: What do you mean I got scared!

READER: I think you couldn't handle the feelings of helplessness and rage Maria's story elicits, and felt uncomfortable about defending her family. So you were forced to add a note of hope.

AUTHOR: Now I know what I've suspected all along—you are a psychologist. But I won't hold it against you. You're probably right.

READER: You should call the piece "Anatomy of a Murder, by Salvador Minuchin." You're full of reinterpretation.

AUTHOR: I don't think I introduce complexities just for aesthetic pleasure. As a matter of fact, the piece owes a lot to a paper I read a number of years ago, by Erving Goffman. It was about an employee who developed paranoid ideas. His coworkers at the office responded to his behavior by distancing themselves, talking about him in private but quickly breaking off the conversation if he came near, avoiding his eyes: exhibiting in full a behavior that validated his sense of persecution. I think the Kepples may have felt like that.

READER: How convenient your "reality" is. Sometimes it's a mere psychological construct. But when you're indulging your interest in context . . .

AUTHOR: You're right, both times. But I think I am too. When you think systemically, reality is multifaceted, depending both on the context and on the position of the observer.

READER: All right, what about your foster-family-care idea? Has it ever been tried?

AUTHOR: Of course. By the Minuchin family, and probably millions of others. But formally—only once, to my knowledge. An agency won a grant to establish such a project, but they got so stuck in the bureaucratic ways of the Department of Welfare that ultimately they simply returned the money. It's quite a story. But I still think the idea is a good one.

Parent Murder

Pierre Rivière

I, Pierre Rivière, having slaughtered my mother, my sister, and my brother, and wishing to make known the motives which led me to this deed, have written down the whole of the life which my father and my mother led together since their marriage. I was witness of the greater part of the facts . . . as regards the beginning I heard it recounted by my father when he talked of it with his friends and with his mother, with me, and with those who had knowledge of it. I shall then tell how I resolved to commit this crime, what my thoughts were at the time, and what was my intention.

This is the beginning of a strange document, written in 1835 by a French peasant who had just committed the triple murder he describes. Pierre Rivière's *Memoir,* a history of the trial, the indictment, contemporary medical opinions, and other relevant documents, were published in 1973 in a book edited by Michel Foucault, *I, Pierre Rivière.*

I read the book after studying the case of Maria Colwell and was struck by the symmetry of the two cases. Maria was murdered by her stepfather. Pierre murdered his pregnant mother and two of his siblings (a reminder that violence in families is not solely a parental prerogative). The commentaries on the two are also similar. The Crown's inquiry into Maria's death focused on a safety net geared to the individual child so exclusively that it failed to save her. The legal-psychiatric controversy of Pierre's time focused on the murderer's mental state. A century later Foucault and his associates provided a sociocultural analysis of the case. In both cases the organism that mediates between the child and society—the family—is overlooked.

Pierre himself devoted two thirds of his memoir to his family. What happens when you look at Pierre with a focus on that family? The murders remain; everything we know about Pierre was gathered in that light. As with Maria Colwell, we know who did it. But we don't know what did it. What was the geography of the act? Who were the murderer's accomplices? And how did his victims attract the lightning?

Pierre's *Memoir* was written at the request of the magistrate, but it had been mentally drafted before the murders as a careful justification of the action. Foucault viewed it as a description but also as the spring that propelled the act. "He contrived the engineering of the narrative/murder as both projectile and target, and he was propelled by the working of the mechanism into the real murder. And, after all, he was the author of it all in a dual sense: author of the crime and author of the text." For me, it is Pierre's description of his family that is of interest, for it reconstructs the context of that act of violence.

Summary of the tribulations and afflictions
which my father suffered at the
hands of my mother
from 1813 to 1835.

My father was the second of the three sons of Jean Rivière and Marianne Cordel, he was brought up in honesty and religion, he was always of a mild and peaceable disposition and affable toward all, and so was esteemed by all who knew him.

Unfortunately, Pierre's estimable father, Pierre-Margrin Rivière, was eligible for the draft—a dangerous situation in 1813. He therefore set about the task of exempting himself. Through one François le Comte at Courvaudon, he asked for the hand of Victoire Brion. Six months later "they went to sign the contract in the presence of Maître Le Bailly, notary at Aunay. The clauses of this contract stipulated that husband and wife should have a joint estate comprising all movable property and immovable property present and future."

From that original contract until the dissolution of the family twenty-one years later, Pierre describes the transactions between his parents as a succession of conflicts in which contracts and litigations about breach of contract occurred in a constant stream.

Problems began almost immediately: "on their marriage night they did not bed together, because the recruiting board had not yet arrived, and my mother said: he has only to get me with child and then leave, and then what will become of me? As this was reasonable, my father did not compel her to bed with him." Instead, Pierre-Margrin returned to his home at Aunay, while the bride returned to her parents at Courvaudon. For most of their marriage, the couple kept to the two households, the father living with his parents, an aunt, and an uncle at Aunay, and the mother living with her parents at Courvaudon.

Pierre was born in 1815. He was followed by Victoire (1816), Aimée (1820), Prosper (1822), Jean (1824), and Jule (1828). The children, like the properties, became the subjects of endless quarrels.

> I was living with my father at Aunay. I was three or four years old, my mother came with her mother to fetch me, she found me in the meadow where they were haymaking . . . without saying a word to anyone she took me and carried me off. As I cried out my father ran after her, and said he would not let her carry me away . . . My mother . . . started screaming in the streets: I want my child back, I want my child back, and she went straight to the cantonal judge at Villers to ask him whether my father had the right to keep her child from her.

The children were part of the assets of the Rivière-Brion marriage and were apportioned out as such. The couple's legal battles around the fulfillment of contracts included the possession of the children as well as the properties. Accordingly, the children alternated between the two households. But by the time of the murder in 1835, Pierre, Aimée, Prosper, and Jean were members of the father's household at Aunay. Victoire and the youngest child, Jule, were in the mother's camp at Courvaudon.

Each side of the family demanded close proximity and stringent loyalty, which included constant attacks on the other side and attempts to seduce the children of one side to join the other. Pierre-Margrin and Victoire Brion continued to live as members of their respective families of origin, to which they added their children, and the children grew up as members of competing systems. In 1835, the Rivière family looked like this:

Aunay	*Courvaudon*
Paternal grandfather (dec. 1826)	Maternal grandfather (dec.)
Paternal grandmother	Maternal grandmother (dec.)
Aunt	
Uncle (dec.)	
Pierre-Margrin Rivière .... Victoire Brion*	
Pierre	Victoire*
Aimée	Jule*
Prosper	
Jean (dec.)	

* Murdered by Pierre, June 3, 1835

The continuity of life within the two extended families prevented the development of the couple as a separate subsystem.
The Rivière nuclear family never had a chance. In fact, it is
tempting to call the Rivières an "open lineage system" rather
than a nuclear family. But they lived in a nineteenth-century
Catholic society in which the patriarchal nuclear family was the
norm. Pierre felt that kinfolk, neighbors, priests, magistrates, and
God himself watched in horror the unnatural determination of
Victoire Brion not to submit to her lawful husband and master.

Pierre, who helped Pierre-Margrin work both farms, was his father's devoted son. In the *Memoir* Pierre-Margrin is unfailingly
presented in terms of Christian meekness and resignation. Victoire Brion is invariably in the wrong, even in the quarrels within
her own clan.

> I saw that the quarrels between my [maternal] grandmother and
> mother were still going on, but my mother got the upper hand over
> my grandmother who was growing feeble, this poor good woman was
> completely miserable, not only did she suffer from the continued
> quarrels, but several persons reported having seen my mother strike
> her and drag her by the hair.

The quarrels between the father and mother escalated, growing
increasingly violent, and family members took positions in the
conflict. A number of cross-generational coalitions were formed:
grandmother, father, and son against wife; grandmother, mother,
and daughter against father. These coalitions sometimes shifted
within the clan. There were also attempts by the parents to re-
cruit allies from the other camp. Pierre describes an attempt by
his mother to gain the loyalty of her daughter Aimée by describ-

ing an affair she said the father had with another woman.

The transactions of running the farms became constant areas of conflict between husband and wife. They quarreled about the buying and selling of land, the houses, and the cows. The mother accused the father of not giving her the money she wanted to start a store. He countered that she was incurring unnecessary expenses in order to bring his financial ruin, and so on and on. Pierre's descriptions of these quarrels are interesting because he often describes incidents in which he could not have been involved. This may be the product of his fantasies; he may have brought delusions to the justification of his crime. But more probably he is quoting Pierre-Margrin's descriptions of his struggles with his wife, confided to Pierre as ammunition in the war of coalitions, father and son against wife and mother.

In 1833 Pierre's maternal grandmother died, and Pierre's mother became the head of the Courvaudon household. After twenty years of marriage, the father now insisted that the mother join him at Aunay. They agreed that mother would move to Aunay and they would rent Courvaudon. Pierre and his father came with a cart to take some furniture from the house, and the usual conflictual dance reappeared:

> My father asked for the key of a loft and when [my mother] refused he took a chest which was in the house, my mother objected; then he held her while I loaded it with the man who was with us. As he held her she set to scratching his face and bit him in several places, my little brother Jule coming up, she told him: bite him, bite that wretch ... but seeing that the child was worrying him I caught hold of him and carried him into a neighboring house, we finished loading and went off. In the afternoon we went back, as we arrived the whole village came out of their doors, my mother set to arguing, and my father climbed in a window to get into a loft, then she seized him by the legs and pulled him down, broke his watch-chain and tore his clothes, he did not strike her at all, but he said he would shut her up in a house to keep her quiet, he caught hold of her to carry her away, but her hands were free and she scratched him again even worse than the first time, then he seized her hands to take her into that house and she fell down purposely; he did not drag her, as she said, but he tried to get her on her feet to take her there, my sister joined in to stop my father, and seeing that she was hindering him, I pulled her away and slapped her several times while my father took my mother off, she was shouting

and so was my sister: vengeance, he is murdering me, he is killing me, vengeance, my god vengeance.

Nonetheless, the mother moved to Aunay, uniting the family for the first time under one roof. But the conflicts did not cease.

Since their great quarrels my father had had no carnal intercourse with her. Nevertheless if only to enrage her he wanted to try on the first or second night. My sister Victoire heard. Then she said: oh my god my god what are you doing to her? Look you, he said to her, what business of yours is it, I am doing to her what men do to their wives; ah, she said, let her be since she does not want it . . . He bedded with her several nights and then seeing that she did not leave him any feather cover on his side or feathers in the pillow, and she was doing all she could to cause mischief, he preferred to sleep in the other bed, and my sister and my brother ever after bedded with my mother.

The mother decided to separate again. She took the father to court and, as a condition of their marriage contract, demanded that he give back furniture, money, and cattle. The mother won these legal battles (probably because the judge wanted to avoid her importunities, in Pierre's opinion). Pierre became greatly concerned about his father, who was making suicidal threats. He began to form his plan, the solution to his father's problems.

I read . . . a history of shipwrecks . . . I found in it that when the sailors lacked victuals, they sacrificed one of their number and ate him to save the rest of the crew. I thought to myself: I too will sacrifice myself for my father, everything seemed to invite me to this deed.

So on June 3, 1835, he dressed in his Sunday clothes and asked Aimée to sing the canticle "Happy Day, Holy Joy." Then he took a pruning hook and murdered his mother, Victoire, and Jule. "I have just delivered my father from all his tribulations. See that my father and my grandmother do not do themselves a mischief," he told some passing neighbors. "I die to restore them peace and quiet." Pierre hid in the woods and fields for a month, but was finally arrested and arraigned. And now the second part of his history begins, the reaction of contemporary experts to his case.

Pierre as the Criminal Patient

A local physician examined Pierre and read his *Memoir*. He came to the conclusion that Pierre was essentially normal and that the triple murder could be ascribed "only to a state of momentary overexcitement brought on by his father's tribulations." But the psychiatrist called in by the defense, Dr. Vastel, labeled him a monomaniac. The jury found Pierre guilty of parricide but suggested a request for clemency from the king. At the end of the year, five of the most important psychiatrists in Paris read the report of Dr. Vastel, Pierre's *Memoir*, and various legal documents. They signed a report concluding that Pierre was insane.

The death sentence was commuted by the king, and Pierre was sentenced to life imprisonment in the central prison at Beaulieu. He hanged himself there four years later, on October 19, 1840.

The Verdict: Pierre in Context

To the government, press, lawyers, psychiatrists, and newspaper readers of Pierre's own time, the overriding question was of course: Was Pierre sane? If the crime were committed today, the reaction would be the same. Prosecution, defense, and examining doctors would zero in on his *Memoir*, now as then, on the few pages Pierre included to explain his character by focusing on incidents in his own life. His fantasies, play relationships with peers, feelings of being different, dreams of great deeds—the life of a very lonely child—remained the juicy data on which psychiatrists were to build a psychopathological nosography. But Pierre himself devoted two thirds of the *Memoir* to his family, to the context of his violent act. Many people, both psychotic and functional, have destructive fantasies that are never projected into action. What was the context that impelled Pierre Rivière to murder?

Like our own period of technological revolution, Pierre's postrevolutionary world was permeated with violence. Several of his uncles were killed in the wars that had endured almost continuously for a quarter of a century, and Pierre was born in the year of the final defeat at Waterloo. The regime of Louis Philippe brought comparative stability, but episodes of random violence were common throughout France during the years of Pierre's lifetime. Within the Rivière-Brion family, violence was the constant companion of family interaction. It was also a method of demonstrating loyalty. A violent loyalty bound Pierre-Margrin and Victoire Brion to their own families. That became the glue that bound Pierre to his father's subsystem. In the end, the triple murder was also an act of loyalty, the fealty of a member of a subsystem to the leader of that coalition.

For Pierre, a lonely and marginal child, there seemed to be no life outside the family. The conflicts between his parents became the focus of his observations and fantasies. He developed incest fantasies and phobias toward women, which were reinforced by his religious fanaticism and his conclusion that history proved the tyranny of women over men was unnatural.

> It is the women who are in command now in this fine age which calls itself the age of enlightenment . . . I thought it would be a great glory to me to have thoughts opposed to all my judges, to dispute against the whole world . . . I said to myself: that man [Bonaparte] sent thousands to their death to satisfy mere caprices, it is not right therefore that I should let a woman live who is disturbing my father's peace and happiness.

> I wholly forgot the principles which should have made me respect my mother and my sister and my brother, I regarded my father as being in the power of mad dogs or barbarians against whom I must take up arms.

What voices are we hearing? The closed world of the Rivière family, with its suspicion against the outside, against established institutions, the judges, the church, the king. Pierre-Margrin and Pierre's feeling that Victoire Brion always won expanded into a war of the sexes, in which Victoire's death would be a blow for man: "I thought that an opportunity had come for me to raise myself, that my name would make some noise in the world . . . and that in time to come my ideas would be adopted and I should be vindicated." The narrow world of Pierre's family, with its petty conflicts, its litigations, its demand for loyalty, and its aggressive competitiveness, was transformed by Pierre through a quixotic distortion into killing the "maid" to save the "king."

But these fantasies evolved slowly—not in isolation but in dialog and action. Pierre, a triangulated son, participated in the parents' battles, always carrying the father's banner. He struck his sister Victoire and his brother Jule while his father immobilized his mother. He was, like his sister Victoire, a witness of his mother's rape, and each sibling defended the parental ally. The violence in the family was always carried out in the presence of and with the support of the whole clan.

Let me indulge in a fantasy. How would I work with the Rivière family today? They would be different today, of course, and they would probably be referred by a priest concerned with Pierre's odd behavior or by a social worker concerned with the violence between the parents. In any case, I would start by interviewing each subsystem separately. My entrance, as always, would be an attempt to join with each one of the family members in ways that would help them to see me as relevant in the situation. I would listen respectfully to their reality and, while confirming it, would question their experience, suggesting alternative realities that are available and hopeful. In the process I would learn their language and begin to sharpen it.

As part of a natural pattern for the Rivières, each subsystem would try to convince me of the correctness of its unique perspective and try to enlist me on that side. The pull would allow me to understand the emotional and intellectual impact of the family blueprint on its members. I would create scenarios whereby I could see the family members enacting their usual dance. I would ask the young Victoire to talk with the grandmother and would see the mother's intrusion in this dialog; I would ask Aimée to talk with Pierre or with the father, and would comment on interruptions by the third member; I would support the children's loyalty to the family in such a way that they would question it.

After two or three sessions with each subsystem, I would request a meeting of the total family, but would try to induce the grandmothers into the position of observers, along with me, of the family's behavior. In these sessions I would ask the parents to talk with each other and observe the enactment of the coalitions: Pierre/Prosper/father/Aimée/paternal grandmother, or mother/maternal grandmother/Victoire (I would probably ask little Jule to remain home during the first interview with the two subsystems). I would casually begin to block attempts at "help" by the members of the coalition, using humor, and most probably authority, to suggest that the help is unhelpful or disrespectful, or whatever is meaningful in their value systems. Probably helpfulness, loyalty, and fairness were important in the Rivière family.

Then I would activate the sibling subsystem, trying to move the focus toward Pierre and Victoire, using Aimée or Prosper as my "cotherapist." I would point to the ways in which they fight out disagreements that are not their own but their parents'—how they are puppets or shadows. Probably I would express my amazement at the fact that Pierre, though he is very intelligent, uses only his father's brain and not his own, and I would audibly wonder why. In the process I would highlight each family member's strength, becoming a source of their enhanced self-esteem. Pierre and young Victoire would get my full support and a challenge as well. I would support their individuality, talents, possibilities, and would challenge their narrowness—but I would absolve them of it, since the responsibility for their childishness lies in their parents' request for help and in their fantastic loyalty. But immediately I would go to the parents' rescue, construing the children's attempts to help as disrespectful of their own strength and possibilities. I think it would be possible to get Pierre and Victoire to form a coalition against the parents' control, since coalitions against somebody were certainly possible steps in the family dance. Joining Pierre and his sister in a pas de deux would normalize Pierre and pull him toward a world of communication with peers.

At this point, my fantasy stops. What then? Probably they would indicate my way. The Rivières of this world come with different voices, but they are more or less willing to teach the willing therapist, if the therapist first convinces them of his relevance to their plight and brings along a pouch full of possible realities. The sessions would sometimes carry an element of violence, but in the many years of my work with families having delinquent adolescents, I have rarely found myself in a situation that I could not control with words or with an orderly withdrawal. I think that family violence should be treated with family healing. Only when you remove the violence from a family member, and locate it in the interactions among the members, can you determine the appropriate distance for defusing destructiveness.

As for madness and responsibility, the concept of "not guilty for reasons of insanity" is a legal, not a psychiatric, concept. *After* the murders, it seemed important for the medical-legal establishment of the time to determine Pierre's degree of responsibility. And they were correct in their findings: Pierre was mad. But clearly, as

Foucault's analysis points out, he was quite sane and talented as well. From our perspective, we can see that the organism of Pierre/Pierre-Margrin/Victoire Brion was violent and mad (and that Pierre in this context was psychotic), while the organism of Pierre/Aimée/paternal grandmother was sane (and Pierre, as part of that pattern, was sane).

When we look at Pierre in his family, we begin to understand to what extent his act of violence was an extension of the violence of his time, his society, and his family. Within this context, murder seemed the logical solution to the impasse of two systems that could neither integrate nor, because of their economic interdependence and the legal situation, separate. When Pierre finally killed himself, he was only putting the correct ending to a story in which acts of violence were the affirmation of one's loyalty.

READER: Intervening in a nineteenth-century family? It has the merit of originality, I suppose. And I confess I'm intrigued by your diagnostic categories. Pierre/father/mother is psychotic. But isn't a diagnostic system of this kind extremely unwieldy?

AUTHOR: Certainly. For simplicity, we have to return to the individual apart from context—which always reminds me of the drunk who lost his keys in the middle of the street but went to look for them at the corner because there was a light there. Our tendency to impose order on life simplifies things, but it also distorts.

READER: But how can you treat a process without identifying it?

AUTHOR: I thought I identified the process of violence by locating it in a specific threesome. That seems to offend your sense of order.

READER: I'm not concerned with order. I want to know who was responsible.

AUTHOR: So do I.

READER: Pierre's mother was one of his victims. He killed her. Are you ruling her death suicide against all the evidence?

AUTHOR: The evidence of Pierre's *Memoir* argues that it was suicide—as well as murder of course.

READER: There you go again. When violence is committed against a person, there should be a clear separation of the criminal and the victim.

AUTHOR: It's not so easy when you deal with families. As you saw, I have actually had to invent a diagnosis: "anorectic family," even though anorexia nervosa is clearly a disease of one individual.

READER: The perpetrator of a violent act should be held responsible for that act.

AUTHOR: I think I understand your confusion. You're concerned with the act of violence and retribution—possibly reparation. This is the judicial system's position. I am concerned with understanding—and therefore possibly preventing—the violent act. That is what the mental-health system should be doing: identifying the context of potential violence before it is enacted.

READER: From your point of view, we should revamp the entire relationship between the judicial system and mental health.

AUTHOR: Yes. We should.

An Alternative

Violence and Healing

Lars and Astrid Andersson's fourteen-year marriage was marred by recurring episodes of violence. When sober, Lars was cooperative, gentle, and rather shy. Under the influence of alcohol he could explode. Astrid and their fourteen-year-old daughter Sonja lived in fear of these outbursts. About six weeks before this interview, Astrid celebrated her thirty-second birthday. At her party she told Lars to get out the "adult" videotape they'd bought in Sweden, to lend it to her sister and brother-in-law. Lars did as he was told, but in bed that night he kept his hand on Astrid's throat, threatening to choke her to death, and he forced sexual activity on her.

Astrid went to a women's shelter to explore her legal options. They offered to help her file for separation. Instead she returned home, and the family life continued as before. Her doctor prescribed a tranquilizer to calm her, but she suffered "nervous" seizures that left her trembling on the floor. The following week Sonja came home six minutes past the established family curfew. Lars decided the appropriate punishment was to slap her one time for every minute she was late. Before the sixth slap Sonja tried to stop him: "If you do that again, I'll never forgive you!" Infuriated, Lars made the sixth slap a real blow; Sonja fell and hurt her ear. She had to be hospitalized and was told there is a possibility of permanently reduced hearing in that ear.

I have deliberately used neutral language to describe two episodes of violence in the Andersson family. In real life, they were full of pain, rage, and helplessness. But the Anderssons impressed me as genuinely nice people—a trifle naive, perhaps, but Lars and Astrid cared for each other and for their daughter. I liked them and they liked me, and there's the rub: in the abstract, I hate men who abuse children or rape women. I have a strong feeling of discomfort when I read about such cases. At times I have startled my wife with my primitive notion that castration may be a proper social response and deterrent to rape, certainly not the measured response of a scientist. How could I understand Lars, or Astrid for that matter? Why did they continue a marriage with such destructive patterns? Equally important, how should we respond when we are called, as professionals, to intervene in such situations?

As a systemic thinker, my view is that transactions among family members follow an elliptical pattern. Any act is a midpoint—a response and a stimulus in a series of recursive loops. But how does this theoretical model with its logical determinism apply to people like the Anderssons? Lars raped his wife, there is no doubt of that. He sent Sonja to the hospital, and her loss of hearing is a direct consequence of Lars' sixth slap, not a midpoint in a recursive loop. Yet if we focus on the violent act, how can we intervene?

Lars and Astrid could separate, except it seems that neither of them wants that. Sonja could be removed from their care to the problematic safety of an institution or foster care, leaving her bereaved parents permanently labeled as abusing and ineffective. Lars could be prosecuted or, less harshly, watched. But this is intervention with a bludgeon. Unquestionably something must be done. Continuing in the same way is not the answer; nor are the denial and concealment so often characteristic of both alcoholism and family violence.

Feminist advocates have responded to situations like this by developing refuges where battered wives find protection from husbands' brutality and, more important, a community of concerned women ready to help them break the patterns that keep them trapped as victims. Some groups attempt the difficult job of increasing male and female awareness of the way our culture controls and narrows our responses. But many of these refuges maintain a policy that keeps their doors closed to men, not only the abusing relatives but any other variety, including males of the "helping professions." This is again a solution that dismembers.

In a powerful book about incest and sexual abuse of children (*I Never Told Anyone*), men and their victims are described as the product of our culture.

Men are taught to equate power and violence with a sense of well being. Many seek this sense of well being so desperately, so recklessly, that they are willing to look for it even in the bodies of children. Their concern for the child is too weak to check them, their desire for domination too strong.

A little girl can be used sexually because she is property, or because she is biologically imperfect, or because she is an enticing, sexy temptress . . . If she is violated, the culturally imposed concept of her sexuality renders her culpable. Any attempt on the part of the child to expose her violator also exposes her own alleged inferiority and sexual motives and shames her rather than the offender.

The editors of this book draw from a series of terrible stories of male destructiveness a program aimed at making children and women able to resist male destructiveness. I sympathize with their view. But I think that, like the British court, their epistemology and therefore their actions maintain and support what they attack. Focusing on the male as monster makes people experience their individual separation, and perpetuates defensive aggression as a response to aggression. The goal should be to explore and improve people's interdependence.

But let us return to the Anderssons. Astrid went back to Lars, as described. But declaring that his actions were the last straw, she brought him to a family therapy clinic in Oslo. The family had been in therapy for about a month when I came to the clinic as a visiting lecturer. The Andersson's therapist, Irene Levin, suggested a session with the family. It was conducted in Norwegian, with Levin acting as both therapist and interpreter (the translation interpositions have been omitted for this book). Astrid and Sonja understand English and speak it to some extent; occasionally they threw in a word. The staff of the institution watched from behind a one-way mirror, where my wife and coteacher, Pat, provided an ongoing analysis of the session.

We began with the whole family together, focusing on the communication of father and daughter. The accustomed pattern quickly appeared. Their contact was both uncomfortable and rather inept. They lapsed into long silences, which activated Astrid. Soon Sonja was speaking exclusively to her mother. Even if Lars directed a comment to Sonja, Sonja would answer Astrid, and Astrid would convey Sonja's response to Lars. The subject matter seemed simple enough: Sonja wanted a minibike. It seemed that all her friends had one. That was precisely Lars' objection: he "didn't care for that bunch."

The therapeutic point of entry, of course, was not the disagreement, but the observation that somehow Lars and Astrid had agreed that rearing a daughter was a mother's job. Accordingly, the first half of the session was devoted to exploring possibilities in the father/daughter dyad and blocking Astrid from stopping their transactions. I chatted with Sonja in a friendly, nonjudgmental fashion, modeling that possibility for Lars, then got them to talk together, recruiting Astrid to join me *as an observer,* to see whether they could learn to communicate. Their discussion was stilted but positive, and made it possible to assign a task: teaching each other about themselves. Sonja had a lot to learn about men; Lars could teach her. Lars obviously knew very little about young adult women. Could they enlarge each other's horizons?

It seemed obvious that Lars's violence toward his daughter was not (as is sometimes the case) a matter of proximity, but rather of distance—a sense that he could not make contact with his own child. This was related to the wife's position between them as well as to his lack of skill. So I drew Astrid in as my cotherapist. With Astrid's permission, could Lars and Sonja spend an hour—no longer—together three times during the coming week, telling each other something about themselves? I obtained Astrid's permission, and her promise that she would not interfere. In turn, I assured her that nothing violent would happen. Sonja was sent home, with her parents remaining.

This summary doesn't describe the difficulty of the process. The actual session involved a rightfully angry adolescent, a rightfully angry mother, and a defensively silent father. To break that pattern, I had to join with each of the family members, confirm and support them, inspire confidence, promote and accept their dependence on me, introduce "magical" material (like my sureness in predicting future behavior), keep the lid on the women's anger, and fan the family members' wish to cooperate in the process of change.

This approach might be seen as a form of copping out—letting the man off the hook and dismissing his destructive behavior with a shrug. I see it as the only rational way of dealing with family violence. By now my bias should be obvious. I cannot support family maintenance when the family organization is destructive to its members. The goal then is to help the family separate. But if the family wants to continue as a family unit, and if I find this feasible, I must accept my responsibility to help the family change.

It took all my skills as a convincer to organize this task. All of the family members were in foreign territory, and I had perched myself on a rather precarious limb. Assuming responsibility for the task and a positive outcome was an act of faith in systems theory. My experience of the Anderssons in the first part of the interview told me they were nice people, but violence can occur in families of nice people. What triggers it, however, is not evil triumphing over good, but a sequence of interpersonal events. I assumed that violence between Lars and Sonja could arise only as a three-person phenomenon, in a context that included Astrid. By creating a context of Lars/Sonja/myself, I felt reasonably certain that violence would not occur. The second part of the interview involved only the couple.

MINUCHIN: Lars, we've talked about things relating to the whole family. But what about your relationship with your wife?

ASTRID: He doesn't realize what's going on. This time he pulled his parents into the battle.

LARS: I didn't pull them in. You did that.

ASTRID: Oh, no. They were there, that's all. This time they saw what's really going on.

LEVIN: What happened? What's the problem?

ASTRID: What happened is that my husband has been drinking even more. A lot more. And he's done a lot of crazy things because of it. That's it in a nutshell. I asked my husband's parents for help. I didn't dare go home to him without having them with me.

LEVIN: Do you agree, Lars? Is that the problem?

LARS: Yes. What she said.

ASTRID: Right before Christmas we decided that you could have just two drinks a day. But you broke that promise. Then after we started in therapy we decided, right here, that you shouldn't drink at all. But you—

LEVIN: What was the final agreement?

LARS: That I shouldn't drink.

ASTRID: I tell you I can't take it any more! I start shaking as soon as I see a bottle.

LEVIN: Did you agree, Lars?

LARS: Yes. Well, we decided.

M: What makes you drink? Wait, Irene. Let me put that better. How does your wife make you drink?

Astrid felt comfortable challenging Lars's violence to Sonja. Alone with him, she has changed tactics and is attacking only his drinking. This is a focus that excludes interpersonal confrontation: Lars's need for control, his demands that Astrid submit, and his physical violence all disappear, and the only remaining issue is his drinking. Drinking is a conflict area where the couple can complain about each other endlessly with no demand for change. I'll have to challenge this defensive maneuver. But in order to do that I must first travel with them along their worn path: his drinking and her control over his drinking.

LARS: I find it very relaxing, one drink. I really do.

M: How does she make you drink? What is there about your relationship that makes you drink?

LARS: I . . . it's not clear. I don't know.

M (to Levin): He has to start thinking about that. He'll stop drinking only when he knows what Astrid is doing that makes him drink. Think together.

ASTRID: You feel it as a defeat if I say that I'll leave you if you drink. I said last weekend that you've got to choose: me or the bottle. But he'll feel it as a defeat if he doesn't get both.

Astrid is right. But her solution is still confined to "He's got to stop drinking."

LARS: No! I've got to decide by myself.

M: You're close to understanding, but you still don't understand.

LARS: If I understood, there wouldn't be any problem.

ASTRID: But you understand how nervous I get when you drink. A lot of negative things have happened while you were drinking.

Astrid and Lars are displaying, paradigm-perfect, one of the dynamics common in families with an alcoholic member. Wife or husband begs spouse not to drink. Drinker agrees not to drink, feeling controlled by spouse, and consequently disowns the drinking. But drinker continues to drink, now under the rubric, "s/he can't tell me what to do." Husband or wife begs spouse not to drink, and so on.

LARS (*gently*): You've always been nervous.
ASTRID: Because of you!
LARS: What do you mean because of me? Is there some connection between your damned nerves and—
M: How long have you been married?
ASTRID: Fourteen years.
M: And you still don't see the connection?

Through the years Lars's drinking has become the "cause" of all family problems. This fixing of causality on the behavior of one person blurs the nature of the other family transactions. Lars is not free to resent Astrid's behavior, since he is forced to admit that he is the cause. But because he feels that he is not really the cause, that he doesn't drink all that much, and that she's just seizing the opportunity to keep him in the doghouse, he drinks to prove that he is treated unfairly, that he is independent, that he has the right to his own life, that he is a man. The goal in this situation is to have the drinker take possession of his drinking, own it and see it as his, so that controlling it becomes a matter of personal competence and control rather than a knuckling under. But, paradoxically, an effective means to this end is to emphasize complementarity: "How does your wife make you drink?" Bringing the drinking into the interpersonal arena can open both the drinking and all sorts of overshadowed marital issues to productive exploration.

M: You need to think together. What does she do that makes you drink?
ASTRID: I've asked myself that so many times. What do I do to

make you drink? I asked you this weekend. Am I too strong? Do I talk too much? But you don't allow me to do anything either! This is absolutely your last chance!

The pattern has just been repeated. Wife threatens, husband tests. It is as remorseless and unending as a piston.

M: Will you really leave him if he drinks? Or will you do as you have always done?

ASTRID: I will leave him!

M: Are you sure?

ASTRID: I have no choice. It repeats itself, over and over again. He never changes. And I don't want this any more! He doesn't understand, and it happens again and again. Maybe my nerves are just worse now, but it seems his reactions get worse and worse.

M: Do you want to test her, Lars? Get drunk this afternoon.

LARS: I don't want to do that.

LEVIN: Do you believe her?

LARS: Well . . . I wish I could say no, but I'm not quite sure.

M: She won't leave you.

ASTRID: There's no sense continuing to live in such a relationship. I don't live an independent life anymore. I'm just terrified. Every weekend, every drink . . .

M: But he doesn't believe you'll leave him.

ASTRID: That's because I've said it so many times before. But this time I really . . .

M (to Lars): Get drunk this afternoon. She won't leave you. I can guarantee that. She won't leave you.

The Anderssons are familiar with their own pattern. They've played it many times through the years. Note that there is still no direct interpersonal challenge. She's accusing him of drinking, of abusing his daughter, of making her life miserable. But there is no request for change in interpersonal transactions, only that he stop drinking.

ASTRID (to Levin): Why does Minuchin think I'm so dumb? Why wouldn't I leave him? A relationship that gives me enormous nervous problems . . . why should I continue to destroy myself? Because I'm sure now that's really happening. And another thing, I can't continue to stand between my husband and my daughter. I see now—

Astrid is diffusing my impact, reestablishing the familiar pattern, this time attacking me instead of Lars. My strategy would force husband and wife to confront each other. Astrid is avoiding that, as she has for fourteen years, with a shrapnel defense.

M: Lars, do you feel your marriage is satisfying?
LARS: Yes.
M: Can you see ways that your life could improve if your wife changed a little bit?
LARS: Yes. Well, not that she changes. But maybe we could understand each other a little better.
M: Tell her the ways you would like her to change.

I am trying to get some specificity into their sense of dissatisfaction with each other. This is going to be difficult, since in spite of their continuous bickering, both Lars and Astrid are habitual conflict avoiders.

LARS: If your nerves would get better, our relationship would get better. I get the feeling I'm not good enough.
M (*to Astrid*): How could Lars help you with your nerves?
ASTRID: He has got to see clearly—in his own eyes—that he can't drink so much!

Back to square one—but this is not surprising. This couple has fourteen years' experience with the same pattern. Furthermore, it would be difficult for any human being to resist grabbing such a demonstrable grievance.

M: You have got to get out of this vicious circle! Astrid, outside of the drinking problem—forget that just for now—what do you want from Lars?
ASTRID: Well, I wish my husband would give me more freedom to go out. I'd like to get out a little bit more. But I feel that he's accusing me when I do.

That's better. Accepting my framework, Astrid is requesting, through me, that Lars change in an area not related to drink. This is different territory, and land I know well—promoting productive conflict. I will try to increase their demands for change, but the demands will have to be kept in interpersonal terms: "Change in this or that area, in ways that will make my life more livable."

M: Good! That's very good, really concrete. Lars, you feel controlled by your wife.
LARS: Yes.
M: She feels controlled by you.
ASTRID: I wish he'd give me more freedom. I can be concrete here too. It's all right for him to go skiing with friends. But I can't even go to an office party on Christmas with my colleagues.
M: Why? What's he afraid of?
ASTRID: I don't know.
M: Ask him.
LARS: You've been out a lot.
ASTRID: That's true, but . . .
M: Ask him.
LARS: I'm afraid she'll play around!

The world of violence is supported by biases. Women are loose, men are animals, communists want to take over the world, Jews control world finances, and some of your best friends are black but would you want your daughter to marry one? In our dichotomies—black and white, man and woman, good and evil, rich and poor, man and nature, light and dark, mountain and climber—we create antagonists where there should be only perspective.

ASTRID: Why do you say that? Have I ever given you the least reason?!
LARS: No. Never.
M: Has she ever been unfaithful to you?
LARS: Never.
M: But you're afraid she will.
LARS: Well—
M: She's a very beautiful woman. You have a lovely wife. Why are you afraid that she'll be unfaithful?

I am provoking Lars, making a slightly seductive contact with his wife, but conveying my own impression that she is desirable but unattainable. This is a promising area.

ASTRID: I'd like to know that too! I've never—!
LARS: I know that. But some time—
M: She wouldn't mean to, but—
LARS: Right.

I like Lars. He is good-natured, friendly, and incredibly narrow-minded. How did this man, so well liked on the job by all his male and female colleagues, develop such foolish notions? This is Norway, in the late twentieth century. In the midst of a culture with remarkably liberal laws, a concerned welfare system that has eradicated poverty, a culture where women have full legal equality, Lars remains Neanderthal man confronting the saber-tooth tiger: Woman and her sexuality.

M: So you don't dare let her go out. How old are you, Astrid?
ASTRID: Thirty-two.
M: And you, Lars?
LARS: Thirty-four.
M: Then why do you treat her like a little girl? Like a six-year-old?
LARS: I don't.
M: Sure you do.
LARS: You've been out many times with your girlfriends, and with men too. Look, it's true I'm afraid something could happen. You think you're up to every trick in the book, but—
M: If you treat her like a six-year-old she really will leave you. She'll have to. You're married to an adult, not a child.
LARS: I don't see that myself. That's something *you're* saying.
M: If you don't let your wife be an adult, she'll have to leave you. She's not a child, or even an adolescent, like Sonja. You have to trust her.
LARS: I do trust her! I let her go out any time.
ASTRID: Not in the last two years.
M (*to Levin*): So. The problem is not only the drinking. He controls his wife. And she controls him.
ASTRID: No.
M: Yes, you control him very much.

ASTRID: I don't—

M: He feels controlled by you.

LARS: That's right. I do.

ASTRID: I don't understand! If he wants to go out with *his* friends, I say—

M: You must understand how you control your husband. He feels controlled by you.

ASTRID: Really?

LARS: Yes, I do.

M: You don't trust him at all. You don't even trust him to talk with his daughter. You think he's a destructive animal. You have to control him because you're afraid he'll blow up. And he has to control you, because if he doesn't you'll play the whore.

To Lars's certainty that "we can call these gentle creatures ours, but not their appetites," Astrid holds her mirror view: men are insensitive animals. For fourteen years their daily transactions have told them the opposite. They have been sensitive to each other's pain and supportive of each other. Each of them has changed, to develop the complementarity of a couple. But in their conflicts, individual bigotry still holds.

LARS: That's not true!

M: Of course it is. That's why you treat her like a six-year-old. You've got to control each other, because Astrid thinks you're an animal and you think she's a whore.

LARS: That's not completely correct.

M: Is it close?

LARS: Well, just playing around doesn't make you a—

M: I exaggerated. You think Sonja may become a whore?

I'm using language like a club. I feel sympathetic to Lars and Astrid, but I also feel infinitely older, or at least more complex. They seem like children caught in a web not of their making. I am the wise old man with the solution to their riddle. By taking their fears and expressing them in gross concrete terms, perhaps I can use absurdity as a midwife for hope.

LARS: No! Not that she'll be a whore. It's true I don't like that crowd she wants to run around with. In a year or two . . .

M (*to Levin*): Are you a whore?

LEVIN: No.

M: Do you believe her, Lars?

LARS: Of course! I don't think she's a—

M: Are you certain?

LARS: Certain? No one can ever be certain. As I know her, as a person, I don't think she's . . . you can never be certain.

Lars has never explored the ramifications of his bias. How many layers of his thinking are contaminated?

M: You can never be certain? Every woman can be a whore?

LARS: No! I didn't say that.

M: You don't trust anybody.

ASTRID: Too right you don't!

LARS: I just trust one person. Me.

M: Do you trust your mother? Is your mother a whore?

I am rather afraid of carrying the inquiry this far. But at this point I know both Astrid and Lars trust me. They know I'm motivated by a wish to help.

LARS: Not as far as I know.

M: But you're not certain. Lars, you must trust your wife. You can trust her. And you've got to demand that she trust you. You are not an animal.

LARS: I don't think of myself as that, anyway.

M: And she's not a whore.

LARS: No she isn't! And I feel that you are using very hard words.

M: She's not a whore. But that's not because you control her. She's her own person. Look at her. She's not a little girl. She's an intelligent woman. Nice looking too. You're a lucky man, but trust her.

LARS: In your heart, you know I trust you.

M (*to Astrid*): Ask him to negotiate some freedom with you. Some way he can show he trusts you. (*To Levin*) If they can change their relationship a little bit, he'll be able to be with his wife without drinking.

ASTRID: I don't expect to be controlled by you! The way you've been these last two years—

M: You need to help him understand women, Astrid. He doesn't understand you, he doesn't understand Sonja, he doesn't understand Irene—he doesn't understand women. How is it that you've been married for fourteen years and he doesn't understand women at all? (*To Lars*) Didn't she teach you anything?

This is one of the ways of helping a couple see the larger pattern. I challenge Lars's control of Astrid, and then when Astrid thinks I'm on her side, I challenge her. Whose side am I on? The couple's. This indicates to both of them that there is a larger consideration.

ASTRID: I think he needs help. I can't help with this.
M: Yes, *you* can teach him about women.

I have challenged Astrid's perspective, indicating that Lars's knowledge of her is formed between the two of them and she is part of the dyad. She rejects this because accepting it would mean accepting conflict.

ASTRID: I'm not sure I'm willing to help any more. I've tried everything I could think of. It didn't help.
M: No, you haven't. You couldn't have, because if he doesn't understand women after fourteen years, it's because you haven't taught him a thing. The way you have related to your husband hasn't taught him to trust you. And you, Lars. Grow up! I've been married for thirty years—my wife's sitting behind that one-way mirror. She's not a whore. And neither is your wife.
ASTRID: Lars, you know I've never—
LARS: I know that. But—
ASTRID: We even had a child. Minuchin is right. How can you think that I'd—
LARS: All right, I'll shut up.
M: Not shut up. Grow up.
ASTRID: And we need help with that. Concrete help.

Astrid's challenge is not only direct; it is unrelated to drinking. She has accepted a role as my cotherapist, dealing with the relationship.

M: You drink because you can't relax at home. And you can't relax at home because your marriage is a marriage of little children. If that changes, you won't need to drink.

I now put the drinking as a symptom of their dyad, instead of the other way around.

LARS: You know I trust you.
ASTRID: No, I don't think so. Why do you always ask me about the men at the office?
LARS: Because I worry about you, that's all. You always think everybody's nice. You don't know.

It will be some time before this is resolved.

M: Is there something you do together that you both enjoy? How about weekends? Could you go out together for about three hours, this weekend?
LARS: Yes, we could go skiing.
ASTRID: No. Skiing? I hate—
M: He wants to go skiing? Do you know how?
ASTRID: Of course I know how. But he always wants to go so fast that I—
LARS: No. That won't happen.
M: If you go skiing together, can you accommodate to your wife's speed? You know women are weak; can you protect her?
LARS: What my wife's talking about is—
M: The issue is that you don't know her, and you don't know your daughter. She doesn't know you; she thinks you're an animal. Before you separate, are you willing to get to know each other?
ASTRID: We need help.

This request is in a different mode. Astrid is hopeful of new possibilities now.

M: Yes, we'll begin with that. For a few hours, this weekend.
ASTRID: If you mean trust him about the drinking, I will not!

But she is afraid of the demand for change that the task carries. She returns to singling out Lars' drinking as the problem. I feel betrayed. I thought that Astrid was willing to chance a new beginning. But of course that was naive. Why should a physically abused woman trust her aggressor's good intentions? After all, I'm only a vendor of possibilities. I won't be there to protect her if he beats her. Still, I know the only hope these two people have is to begin to change their perspective and accept that both of them need to construct their lives. Any dismembering of this organism will only produce a continuation of the same pattern.

M: You haven't understood a word I've said! Not one word! I'm talking about you beginning to trust that your husband is not an animal.
ASTRID: Let him show that.
M (*to Lars*): She's making you drink. She's controlling you, and that's how she makes you drink.

It doesn't matter which side of the coin is up. The direction changes, but not the focus. The goal remains the same: a jump toward a different way of looking, thinking, and experiencing.

ASTRID: But he's much stronger.
M: You are very strong. And you have your daughter and even his parents on your side.
ASTRID: I know that. And if this was the first time, I'd have been willing to reach out to him. But it's happened so many times now.

Astrid naturally wants to feel that the therapist will control this process, directing the couple's change. Without that reassurance, she will find it difficult to enter the task of beginning to trust Lars. And in working with a family in which there is violence, the therapist must take on that responsibility.

M: Irene, tell them you'll help them. But the issue now is that Astrid has to trust Lars, and he needs to trust her. And they have to make good things happen, find pleasure together.
ASTRID: We need help.
M: You will decide this weekend. What can you do—
LARS: I have an idea.
M: Hold it! Decide later.

I stop Lars because I want him to get all the credit for beginning the process of change, outside the therapeutic context. I finish the session by making slightly seductive contact with Astrid again, aimed at changing her orientation toward men and giving Lars the capacity to accept another man's response to his lovely wife.

M: You're a very lovely woman, Astrid. Can you be a lovely woman to him?

ASTRID: Yes.

M: He needs to know something about women.

ASTRID: I feel that we're working against each other.

M: Lars, you need to learn from your wife and your daughter. It's time you learned something about women. (*I rise, to indicate the end of the session. Irene and the couple rise to shake hands. Then, on impulse, I call through the mirror.*) Pat! Can you come in? (*My wife enters the room.*) This is my wife, Patricia. She is a psychologist. And I can assure you, she's not a whore.

Introductions are made all around, everyone smiles and shakes hands. We chat for a few minutes in a social vein; obviously Lars and Astrid are pleased to show their more attractive facets in a couple-to-couple framework. The session ends.

When they returned the following week, Lars and Astrid brought a present for us. It was a Norwegian cheese cutter, and Astrid insisted on demonstrating it on the spot. Lars had spent three hours talking with Sonja, and they enjoyed it. At Lars's insistence, the couple had taken a weekend trip and found the experience new and positive. I have kept in touch with the Anderssons' progress through Irene Levin. They stopped therapy after about four months, but a recent follow-up about eighteen months after this session showed that their improvement has continued. There have been no episodes of violence, and Lars has become only a social drinker.

The quick response of this couple to therapeutic input would indicate that theirs was a case of instrumental violence and that Lars and Astrid were caught in an interaction supported by cultural stereotypes: a culture in which the threat of violence and actual violence were mechanisms that could be used to achieve a goal. In such cases it is frequently possible to change the family's violent patterns by a combination of therapeutic and educational inputs. I don't know what the future holds for the Anderssons. But no one can promise a smooth pathway, only the possibility of new vistas, as humans learn to experience themselves as part of each other. My wife and I cut our Jarlsberg cheese carefully, just the way Astrid showed us.

READER: I liked the case of the Anderssons. That really did seem hopeful. But Maria—Pierre! You're tackling windmills. Do you feel like Don Quixote?

AUTHOR: Impotent, raging, half crazy, and still hopeful enough to dare to charge? Yes, I think that is my mood.

READER: What are your windmills? Hypocrisy? Violence?

AUTHOR: Blinders, I think. We know so much, but we apply our knowledge so poorly. Our chief remedy for violence is a prime example: we control, which engenders violence, which engenders control.

READER: Yes. Your pieces on the court seem to present an impossible dilemma. The protecting interventions themselves continue the cycle of destruction. But not to interfere invites destruction too.

AUTHOR: It's the problem of the blind men, each with one piece of the elephant. We always gerrymander our problems. Urban renewal pushes the poor from one area, solving poverty—in that area. Child abuse requires child protection. Therefore we bring in lawyers, jails, foster homes.

READER: But I see only two possibilities. One is not to intervene in order to avoid the distortion of partial interventions. But that's impossible. Society has to respond when deviation goes beyond an imposed cultural threshold. The other is global change—a kind of Trotskyite universal revolution of ideas. But that's impossible too. Our world is so diverse, with so many cultures—a heterogeneous, pluralistic, cultural soup that . . .

AUTHOR: But to maintain our present forms of response invites the destruction of everything we consider human.

READER: Well, what's your solution? Christian forgiveness? Gandhi's passive resistance? Unilateral disarmament?

AUTHOR: If you think for a moment, you'll realize that what these ideas all have in common is the breaking of pattern. As an un-expected response, they precipitate a crisis in the system and a search for new forms.

READER: Then you *are* talking global revolution.

AUTHOR: Yes and no. Revolution, as humanity has implemented it, has generally resulted in more violence. I'm thinking of the development of crisis.

READER: I think you're playing with words to avoid facing your own confusion and impotence.

AUTHOR: You may be right. I'm in strange waters, being neither a philosopher nor a social planner. But let me tell you what I've learned from watching families: in moments of transition, when families change shape, there is crisis. Old patterns are aban-doned, and new possibilities open that are promising, but vaguely sketched. The compound of hope and insecurity that characterizes families at transitional points seems present in the macrosystem of the world of Pierre, the world of Maria, and the world on the front page of the *Philadelphia Inquirer.*

READER: Isn't it dangerous to try to understand social processes—the dynamics of society—with the observation of small groups like families?

AUTHOR: Yes, certainly. What I am saying is probably wrong from a scientific point of view. But since this is my only per-spective, let me state it. Call it an analogy—a fable or literary license. You remember in "Quartet" I talked about the diffi-culties of a blended family as a shape that does not yet have so-cietal structures to facilitate its development? I think something like this happens when change pulls ahead of human social structures: there is a lack of underpinning. Something like that characterized Pierre's world, the years following the French Revolution. It is a characteristic of our own period of techno-logical revolution.

READER: I take your point. But we did agree that violence is not the necessary product of loss of structure. The violence we are experiencing in our time—

AUTHOR: Is inherent in the dualistic epistemology—the either/or that says only the stronger survives. Violence is inherent in the idea that one must be superior.

READER: That's Darwin's survival of the fittest.

AUTHOR: On the contrary. Darwinian survival of the fittest is not the survival of the stronger, but the survival of the fittest within the environment. It is a concept of cooperation, of interdependence.

READER: Damn! We *do* see with our culture's glasses. And this dualistic position, with technology at its service . . .

AUTHOR: Indeed. The nuclear deterrent is its most horrible metaphor—the ultimate expression of the either/or.

READER: But an ecological perspective, which teaches us we are part of each other, complements—

AUTHOR: It's happening, I think. With the technological revolution, we are also beginning to learn our interconnectedness. As we learn that we are all interdependent, perhaps we can hope for an end to "rugged individualism"—the individualism of the criminal, the cannibal, the conquerer. Perhaps we can learn to see our concepts of self as actually antiself, because they exclude the Other. Perhaps then, at last, we can begin to explore the infinite possibilities of flexibility and cooperation.

READER: We seem to have wandered rather far from the family. Or maybe not. But let me finish with a last question. Do you see any way that family change will help to produce a changed society?

AUTHOR: No. Change is appearing in many independent corners, but it will reach the social field only slowly. Then we will achieve crisis, and a search for new ways. The uncertainties, confusion, and pain that characterize change in the social field will not diminish in our time, but perhaps one day . . .

READER: How will it happen?

AUTHOR: I have no idea. What do you think?

Part Three

Patterns in Context

The Triumph of Ellen West

An Ecological Perspective

> We have yet to write the history of that other form of madness, by which men in an act of sovereign reason confine their neighbors and communicate and recognize each other through the merciless language of nonmadness.
>
> —MICHEL FOUCAULT, *Madness and Civilization*

"Ellen West, a non-Swiss, is the only daughter of a Jewish father for whom her love and veneration know no bounds." This sentence opens "The Case of Ellen West, an Anthropological-Clinical Study," by Ludwig Binswanger, the famous Swiss existential psychoanalyst who was the director of a sanatorium in which this patient was treated. Binswanger based his study not on direct contact with her, but on his readings of her journals and poetry. What we know about "Ellen West" is a psychoanalytic understanding based on the memories she recorded rather than on any knowledge of the living person. Binswanger tells us she was in treatment of one kind or another for half her life. She was seen by two major psychiatrists of her day, Emil Kraepelin and Eugen Bleuler, and by two students of Freud's. Otherwise, she seems to have lived very much as an upper-middle-class European woman. She was well educated, well traveled, passionate about ideas, cultured, and confined. She killed herself at the age of thirty-three, just before the outbreak of World War I.

When I first read the study years ago, I became fascinated with the question of responsibility. Who caused her death, directly or indirectly? Edgar Z. Friedenberg says that her case illustrates "the depth and commitment of existential psychiatry to the client's real sense of herself." Following Binswanger's representation of her as a "living struggle between an authentic and an ersatz form of Being," he cites her suicide as an act of existential courage: "It is better to feel your real selfhood for one fatal day than to go on for years in the ordinary way, trying to carry on metabolism as if one has not died at all." To me, Ellen West became a symbol of the depth of existential psychiatry's commitment to its own conceptualizations. Among many other things, the case of Ellen West is an instance of psychiatrists adhering to their theories.

When I reread Binswanger's essay after working with a number of anorectic families, I became convinced that Ellen West was an anorectic, although that diagnosis appears nowhere in the case records. By then my experience with anorectic families was adding resonance to what I found in her journals and poetry. The result was the play that follows.

The Triumph of Ellen West

Act 1, Scene 1

(Ellen is seated in the middle of the room writing a letter. Her voice is heard as she writes.)

Dear Karl:

   I have been reading my diary. I started writing it when I was fifteen years old, and now it covers eighteen years . . . stepping stones. My first love, a birthday party, a friend's betrayal, a poem to Spring, another to my ugliness, a dried flower marker to a momentous event—what was it?

   You know, today I read a wonderful poem by Rilke. I think he captured the essence of our discussion.

> Narcissus pined. The nearness of his being
> kept on evaporating from his beauty
> like scent of essenced heliotrope. But, seeing
> that just to see himself was all his duty,

(She stops, looks at the audience, biting the pen. At this moment a latecomer, a man in his sixties with white hair and glasses, comes down the theater aisle.)

ELLEN: Sir! Yes, you. The one who just came in.

MEMBER OF THE AUDIENCE (*surprised and embarrassed*): Are you talking to me?

ELLEN: Yes. Could you come here and help me?

MEMBER OF THE AUDIENCE: You mean it?

ELLEN: Yes. I thought it would be nice to have a witness. Would you be so kind? Join me?

MEMBER OF THE AUDIENCE: Well . . . yes, why not? Are you certain? I always wanted to be on the stage. (*He walks up onto stage level, then stands ill at ease, looking at Ellen. She indicates a chair. He sits, facing her.*) What do you want me to do?

ELLEN: Help me look back.

MEMBER OF THE AUDIENCE: I am not a reflective person.

ELLEN: You look like a kind person.

MEMBER OF THE AUDIENCE: Appearances lie; I don't believe in them. I measure. I look at facts. I—

ELLEN: Perfect! I'm lucky today.

MEMBER OF THE AUDIENCE: What's perfect? Why are you lucky today? When did you decide that?

ELLEN: Just now, when I met you. I am trying to expand my past (*she picks up the diary and leafs through its pages*) and see its meaning. I bet you're a judge! Fantastic! Will you hold court?

MEMBER OF THE AUDIENCE: I'm not a judge, actually.

ELLEN: It doesn't matter. You will be. (*She gets up, goes to one corner of the room, and picks up a judge's robe and a wig. She gives them to the man.*) Here you are. Put them on.

MEMBER OF THE AUDIENCE (*puts on the robe and wig; Ellen helps him*): How do I look?

ELLEN: Perfect, Your Honor.

JUDGE: Where do you want to start?

ELLEN: The period of my life before I married, when I still lived with my parents.

JUDGE: And was that period a trial? By the way, what is your name?

ELLEN: Ellen West.

JUDGE: And who was accusing you? Of what?

ELLEN: Of being thin, Your Honor.

JUDGE: Being thin? Who are the accusers?

ELLEN: My parents, Your Honor.

JUDGE: Where are they? If they are the prosecution, they should be in court, shouldn't they?

ELLEN: I will call them, Your Honor (*She goes to a side door and calls.*) Mama! Papa! Please come in. I found a judge.

(*Her parents enter, bringing chairs, and sit together at one side of the stage. Ellen is on the same side, a few yards away. They all look at the judge.*)

PARENTS: Could we start, Your Honor?

JUDGE: By all means. (*To Ellen*) Who is your lawyer? Who represents you?

ELLEN: I will conduct my own defense, Your Honor.

JUDGE: Are you certain you don't want a lawyer? Lawyers know how to say things. You seem too young to know how—

ELLEN: *I* am being accused. I know myself better than anyone else could know me. I also know the accusers. They have been my parents for twenty-eight years.

JUDGE: And you're being accused of . . . what?

ELLEN: Of being thin, Your Honor.

PARENTS: Attempted murder, Your Honor.

JUDGE (*looks from one to the other*): Attempted murder?

PARENTS: Yes, Your Honor.

JUDGE: Where is the lawyer for the prosecution? Who's representing you?

FATHER: We will conduct the prosecution ourselves.

JUDGE (*alarmed*): What? Family cases are very complicated. Wouldn't you prefer to use a lawyer? Lawyers know how to say things.

MOTHER: She's *our* daughter, Your Honor. She's trying to kill our daughter.

JUDGE: I'm confused. Can someone in the court clarify things?

ELLEN: They're accusing me of not eating, Your Honor.

MOTHER: She's killing herself, Your Honor. For the last eight years she's been killing herself slowly.

ELLEN (*to parents*): It's *my* body! You can't control my body. You've controlled my life; you can't control my body.

JUDGE: You cannot accuse them, it's not proper. They have accused you. *They* are the prosecution.

ELLEN: Couldn't I accuse them of . . . of . . . robbing me of my voice?

JUDGE: You're talking. I hear your voice.

ELLEN: Yes, but my voice can't say anything. They took away all the words that make decisions.

JUDGE (*looking at Ellen, then at parents*): So you want to accuse them of . . . grand larceny?

ELLEN: Grand larceny. Yes, Your Honor.

JUDGE (*to parents*): And you want to accuse her of . . . slow suicide?

FATHER: No. Attempted murder, Your Honor.

JUDGE: And who will defend you from your daughter's prosecution?

MOTHER: We will, Your Honor. She has to explain her accusation. We won't feel guilty until proven guilty.

JUDGE: It's a most irregular situation. You are both in the position of being prosecution and defense at once. How do you want to conduct your case? How do you plead?

PARENTS
AND ELLEN: Innocent, Your Honor.

JUDGE: Very confusing. Who will begin? (*To parents*) It seems proper that you start, you're older.

FATHER (*to Ellen*): If you feel we're such bad parents, you can begin with your prosecution.

ELLEN: I didn't say you're such bad parents. It's you who say I'm a disobedient daughter.

MOTHER: And you are. Look at yourself! You're killing yourself.

ELLEN: I'm not doing anything to you. It's *my* body. I just like it thin.

MOTHER: I'll die too.

ELLEN: What?!

MOTHER: If you die, you'll kill me.

ELLEN: That's unfair. It's blackmail!

MOTHER: I'm your mother.

FATHER: You're selecting her over me again. Even if she dies, you should remain with me. I'm your husband.

ELLEN: Now you're fighting over me again. Why don't you fight over someone else's body?

JUDGE: Wait, I don't follow that! You seem like one body with three heads.

FATHER: That's exactly true, Your Honor.

JUDGE: How can I judge you? How can I pass judgment on a part of you?

FATHER: I'm sorry, Your Honor. Should we start at the beginning?

JUDGE: I wonder if anybody or anything could help me with your case. But all right, start where you want.

(*Lights to black*)

Scene 2

(*When the lights come up Father, Mother, and Ellen are seated at the table having dinner. The judge sits in shadow at the back of the stage. Father is polishing his dish with a piece of bread, eating with obvious pleasure.*)

FATHER: The truth is, I'm surprised. It was delicious.

ELLEN: I told you you'd like it.

FATHER: What do you call it, in Italian?

ELLEN: Calamare en su succo.

FATHER: Squid in its juice!

ELLEN: Yes. In Palermo, the vendors cook it in the street. It's very popular and very cheap.

MOTHER: It has a strange consistency—kind of rubbery.

ELLEN: You don't want to admit that you like it.

MOTHER: It's all right, if you don't make a habit of it.

ELLEN: We're too conservative in our taste.

FATHER: And it's your job to expand our horizons?

ELLEN: If you let me.

FATHER: Prepare yourself, Martha. We're going to be reeducated by Ellen. (*To Ellen*) How did you enjoy Sicily?

MOTHER: You look very well. I knew the air of Sicily would do you good.

FATHER: There was nothing wrong with Ellen.

ELLEN: Of course not. But I felt better there.

FATHER: What did you do?

ELLEN: Oh, swimming, walking, visiting small villages, ruins. We went to Mt. Aetna and walked to the top of the volcano. I had a feeling of foreboding. All that pent-up energy . . .

MOTHER: Ellen, sometimes you frighten me. You're so intense. You seem to want so much.

FATHER: There's nothing wrong with her ambition. I wish David had half her drive. (*To Ellen*) You have the enthusiasms I had at your age, and the same will to succeed.

MOTHER: That's not so good, Milton. That's what concerns me. You work so hard, and you don't take care of yourself.

FATHER: Nonsense, Martha. That's your need to mother me. You mother all of us. If you . . .

ELLEN (*interrupting to stop the disagreement*): We went to see some Roman temples. It was a walk of thirty kilometers and Sara didn't want to come, so I went with Frieda. I was in very good shape. When Frieda stopped to rest I went on walking, around and around her, like a satellite to the sun. When we came back I was so hungry I ate a tremendous portion of roast lamb, had a liter of wine, a huge helping of provolone, and topped it off with chocolate cake and cream. Sara and Frieda teased me. I put on over five kilos!

MOTHER: You don't seem plumper to me. As a matter of fact, you seem to have lost weight. (*Passes a tray.*) Don't you want more hazelnut cake? Mary made it specially for you.

ELLEN: No, it's too fattening. Give Father another piece.

FATHER (*reaching for the cake*): Don't make Ellen your garbage can, Martha. I'll have another piece. I have no illusions about my figure. (*Mother cuts the piece in half.*) I rate only half of Ellen's portion?

MOTHER: You're eating too much. You've got to take care of yourself. You know that in your family—

FATHER: What else did you do, Ellen?

ELLEN (*soberly*): I saw poverty. Near the most beautiful scenery, you see children with the big round eyes of hunger. I felt so ashamed of our money, my clothing, my hiking boots.

MOTHER: Where are they?

FATHER: What are you talking about?

MOTHER: Where are your hiking boots? I couldn't find them when I unpacked your things.

FATHER: Why did you unpack her things? She could do it herself.

ELLEN: I gave my boots away and half my clothing. They didn't fit me anyway.

FATHER: A very easy form of socialism—giving away what you haven't earned.

ELLEN: I don't see why you chastise me for doing what you taught me.

FATHER: I like your sensitivity to poverty, but you didn't really share your efforts with them, you shared mine. You will have to produce something before you own the right to revolution.

MOTHER: Your other hiking boots are in your closet, Ellen. They're almost new.

ELLEN (*putting a soothing hand on her mother's arm*): It's all right, Mama. Papa is right. (*To Father*) You're always right. You were right about my engagement to Georges. It was hard to break it off, but you were right to insist that I come home. I think I'm too young for a definite commitment. I'm so easily led. I count on your vigilance—it gives me freedom to experiment in safety.

FATHER (*finishing the cake*): I'm glad you see it that way. I was worried that you might not understand my motives. Mother and I were concerned for your well-being.

ELLEN (*goes to him, kissing him and ruffling his hair*): I know. I know.

FATHER (*pleased by her show of affection he gets up, touches his belly, smoothes his hair*): Well, I've got to get to work. I leave you to share your gossip. Just as long as I'm not the target!

ELLEN: You'll never know!

(*Father leaves. Ellen and Mother remain at the table. Mother speaks as soon as the door closes.*)

MOTHER: I'm so glad you're not angry at Papa. He broke off your engagement for very good reasons.

ELLEN: You know I can only be angry with Papa for a few minutes. As soon as I begin to think, I realize he's right. I'd like to be mad, but in fairness I can't.

MOTHER: He's always thinking about what's best for you. We didn't know Georges, and we couldn't be sure about his feelings for you. Papa's family has a tradition to maintain, and you are somewhat—forgive me—somewhat naive. You're romantic and rich, a good target for adventurers.

ELLEN: Georges wasn't like that! But forget it. I'm home now, where I'm loved and protected. Tell me, how is Papa? (*Suddenly turns to the judge.*) I present this as Exhibit One, Your Honor!

JUDGE (*startled*): What? Have you begun the prosecution?

ELLEN: Yes, Your Honor. I want to emphasize that I was twenty-one years old, of full legal age, when my parents, continuing a procedure they had started earlier, robbed me of Georges.

JUDGE: Are you accusing both suspects or only your mother?

ELLEN: Both of them, Your Honor.

JUDGE: The defendant will return to the dock. Mr. West!

FATHER (*returns and sits by Mother*): You heard her say, with her own voice, "I count on his vigilance to give me freedom (*He pulls a notebook from his pocket and consults a note.*) Yes, it's verbatim—"to experiment in safety." Does that sound like coercion, Your Honor?

MOTHER (*to Ellen*): You were always asking Papa to help you. Do you remember your first year at the gymnasium? You asked him to talk with your history teacher because he gave you a B instead of an A.

JUDGE: This evidence is inadmissible—Ellen was then legally a minor. The clerk will delete this statement from the record, and the jury will clear its memory. (*He hits the sides of his head, first with the right hand, then the left.*) Both left and right brains, please.

FATHER: But I did go, and he changed your mark, and you came and sat on my lap and told me I was the best father in the world.

MOTHER: And he told you that you could always count on him. You said—remember, Ellen?—that to have *us* on your side gave you confidence. I thought you said "us," but you really meant him. You were always closer to Papa.

ELLEN: That's not true. I used to tell you things I never told him. Remember that night I was out with Mark, and I came back at midnight. Papa never knew, because you . . .

FATHER: When was that?

MOTHER: What does it matter, Milton? I knew you'd be angry, and I didn't want you upset.

FATHER: But it made her lose respect for me—and for you too, I think. You're her mother, not her girlfriend.

ELLEN: Stop it! Please, I have a headache.

JUDGE: It's very confusing. For a while I thought I had it, but then it became confusing again. How can I judge who's guilty if you don't stay on your own sides? Proceed, please.

(*Father moves back to join the judge. The lighting changes to spotlight Ellen and Mother, seated again at the table, continuing their conversation.*)

ELLEN: Tell me, how is Papa?

MOTHER: Well, the truth is, he's not very well. With David in the

Clinic, and Sam abroad, and you in Italy, his old fear of getting up in the morning became worse.

ELLEN: Is he worried about his business?

MOTHER: He doesn't discuss business with me. He thinks I wouldn't understand—and he's right, of course. We talk mostly about you children.

ELLEN: So things haven't been good between you.

MOTHER: You know I don't blame him. He's a wonderful husband, but he has this foreboding feeling about life, and with his family upbringing, that's understandable.

ELLEN: What do you mean?

MOTHER: Well, Grandma Rose—you never knew her—she was *the* Jewish Mother. The children were tied to her white skirts. She reminds me of a medieval painting of a Madonna I once saw in Florence—all the people of the town were sheltered under her cloak.

ELLEN: You know, there's always been a bit of a mystery about Papa's family. I know that two of his brothers died young, but . . .

MOTHER (*draws closer, lowering her voice*): That's right. You should know—but don't ever mention it to your father, it would hurt him. Your grandfather was very strict, and the children grew up tied to their mother. She was a gentle person, interested in music and the arts. Did you know that she was a very good pianist? But she was afraid of her husband, and the children became her protectors. She had quiet weeks in which she didn't say a word, and the children would hover around her till she came back to life. They became one unit, grandmother and her six children. Too close—it was difficult for them to separate. Your Aunt Jill had a nervous breakdown the day of her wedding. Uncle Steve shot himself. He was very young—in his twenties. And Uncle Robert committed suicide in a period of sadness. People used to say that to leave Grandma Rose a child had to die or go crazy. But it wasn't so. The other three children married, and they're all outstanding people.

ELLEN: I'm glad you told me. It certainly explains why Papa has been so secretive about his family. And I guess it explains why he pushes and pulls at the same time. He wants us to be independent, but he's always checking on what we're doing.

MOTHER: And you can see why I'm so concerned about him. He's so irritable in the morning, as if some disaster had occurred during the night. I'm always smoothing things for him, making his life predictable. I try to anticipate his fears and his dreams, so that he's always prepared.

ELLEN: Are you replacing Grandma Rose?

MOTHER (*ignoring this*): He was so upset about your engagement to Georges. I was worried—

FATHER (*stands abruptly*): Your Honor! This evidence is inadmissible. It seems directed toward presenting me as a psychiatric case. My daughter and wife seem to have become friends of the court, uniting against me. This is improper, Your Honor. My wife and I—together—are the plaintiffs. I demand that this evidence be stricken from the record.

JUDGE: Motion denied. Your daughter, as the prosecutor, has the right to question your wife about your life, to gather background material for her case. (*To Ellen*) I congratulate you on a most skillful maneuver. I'm beginning to enjoy this case. Please proceed.

(*Lights to black*)

Scene 3

(*The parents and the judge are seated in the background. Ellen is alone in the room, writing in her diary. On the table there are items of food.*)

ELLEN (*reading aloud*): *I'm twenty-one years old and I can't breathe in this atmosphere of hypocrisy and cowardice. I mean to do something great. I'm not thinking of the liberation of the soul. I mean the real, tangible liberation of the people from the chains of oppression. I will make no concessions. The existing order is rotten, rotten down to the core . . . I should like to forsake home and parents and live among the poorest of the poor, and make propaganda for the great cause.* (*Takes a mirror and studies her face, tracing its lines with her finger.*) And who are you, dreaming about revolutions? Hypocritical puppet! Yes, Papa. (*Her voice is high, artificial.*) Yes, Mama. You're right about Georges. It

Note: Speeches in italics are taken from Ellen West's diary, as quoted by Binswanger.

doesn't matter that you don't know him; you have the gift of foresight that only parents have. Who am *I* to question your questions? You will always know better than I what's best for me. Isn't that true, Papa? (*Looking in the mirror, she opens her mouth and pulls the skin of her face down heavily, trying to make it longer and thinner.*) You're a strange creature, Ellen. A chameleon. With Georges, an explorer of new horizons. With Papa, an obedient little girl. Master of many shapes is this Ellen—poet (*making faces in the mirror*), radical revolutionary, meek follower, caring daughter. Lost in a hall of mirrors, is Ellen. (*She gets up and begins to pace.*) No, I don't think they were right. Papa didn't persuade me; he commanded, as if I were one of his business ventures. Would he have acted the same way with Sam or even David? I don't think so. Men have to learn to make decisions and accept responsibility. So you don't command them. You ask, suggest, convince them. But me? Mother must have said (*imitating Mother*), "Milton, I'm concerned about Ellen. She's so young and so impulsive. Ask her to come home." (*Imitating Father.*) "You're right, Martha. I'll write today." And here I am. I didn't resist, didn't even question him. I cried, packed my things, and came home. (*Sits and looks at the mirror.*) Could I have resisted? (*Puffs her cheeks out.*) "I'm twenty-one years old and I love Georges!" But what if they'd given in, and I'd married Georges, and it turned out to be all wrong? (*Sucks her cheeks in, still examining herself.*) I'm putting on weight. What if they're right? And if I ever said to Papa, "You're wrong," could he accept that from me? Mama always protects him. She's so afraid of the suicide that runs in his family. Anyway, who am I to know better than they? (*Looks at her arm, pinches her skin.*) I am putting on weight! Every day I get uglier, imprisoned in fat! (*Continues to study her reflection.*)

JUDGE: Is this evidence in your defense or in the prosecution of your parents? Who's introducing this evidence?

ELLEN   I, Your Honor.

AND PARENTS: We, Your Honor.

JUDGE: I will not permit disturbance in the court! The plaintiffs will approach the bench. (*Ellen and her parents approach the judge.*) Look, we must come to some agreement. This is most irregular. We must have one suspect and one accuser in each scene. I don't mind if you change in the next one, but you are to tell me ahead of time. Is that clear?

ELLEN

AND PARENTS: Yes, Your Honor.

(*Ellen, her parents, and the judge take trial positions.*)

JUDGE: Who is prosecuting now?

ELLEN (*to parents*): This is material from *my* diary.

FATHER: Yes, but you used the last scene with Mother against me.

MOTHER: She tricked me. I didn't know she was going to use it in the trial.

ELLEN: You can't use my material. I can't be forced to present evidence against myself. Isn't that right, Your Honor?

JUDGE: That's true in most cases, but families are very complicated. You never know who . . .

FATHER (*to Mother*): Do we let her present her diary as evidence against us? It's highly subjective material.

MOTHER: Why not, Milton? She's our daughter. If we don't help our own daughter, what good are we anyway?

FATHER: You're right, Martha. Your Honor, we've reached agreement. Ellen will prosecute us this time.

ELLEN: Very well. As you can see, Your Honor, by the time I reached twenty-one I could disagree only in my interior dialogs. My parents had robbed me of my public voice. The process, Your Honor, was so clever that I can't point out the precise moment of the theft. It couldn't have occurred all at once—I would have noticed it. But slowly . . . Probably the first words that disappeared were those expressing dissatisfaction in restaurants, or when we visited relatives or friends. At home I could still express my opinions, so I didn't mind it. Besides, I think one should protect one's family from strangers, don't you, Your Honor? But then it began to happen at home. My father steals in broad daylight, Your Honor. When he gets angry his cheek trembles. (*Points at her father's face.*) Do you notice his tic, Your Honor? It's like a signal, for me to swallow my words. It's like a red flag, Your Honor. If some of my words of disagreement cross that barrier before I can stop them, I lose them forever. My mother's stealing, now—that occurs mostly at dusk. And she suffers when she steals. It's clear she doesn't want to do it, Your Honor. She comes close to me, holds me, strokes me—and when I get up to leave, I notice she has stolen my words to use for distance. Is the evidence clear, Your Honor?

JUDGE: It's admissible in a family court. Your testimony may stand.

FATHER (*stands*): Your Honor, I would like to point out that the prosecution's testimony is based on linguistic analysis, and this is a flimsy science. I could demonstrate, using the same theories, that she controls *our* responses, so that in effect she's producing her own trap.

JUDGE: This is circular thinking, inadmissible in court.

MOTHER (*stands*): But Your Honor—we always finish each other's phrases. We never know who initiated a thought.

JUDGE: Silence. We have agreed to go by the book, one prosecuting, the other defending.

MOTHER: But families are more complicated than that, Your Honor. People are joined . . .

JUDGE: Madam, please do not force me to hold you in contempt. We did agree. It's a simple system: one prosecutes, the other defends. Can you defend yourself without prosecuting the prosecution?

FATHER: It's more complex than that, Your Honor.

JUDGE: Not in my court.

FATHER: Then could we introduce evidence against her if we change scenes? About the way she stole our freedom?

JUDGE: By all means.

(*Lights to black*)

Scene 4

(*Father and Mother sit at the table, which is set for two. They are drinking wine. Ellen and the Judge sit in the background.*)

FATHER: It was the strangest dream. At first I was the Emperor of China, walking slowly through the garden enjoying the pheasants and peacocks. Then the scene changed. There was a feast here at home, and a chef brought me a great silver tray with a silver cover. It had a beautiful design—a lamb roasting on a spit. When he opened the dish, the most delicious smell embraced me. It was *Canard à la paillard.* The duck was stuffed with its own liver and basted in red Italian wine; the chef had added part of the liver crushed with a fork—very much like Mary used to make. Then the dream changed. I was in a Chinese dog cage, placed in the center of the table. You and Ellen were eating large portions of weinerschnitzel, but you were passing me bunches of lettuce through the bars of the cage!

MOTHER (*laughing*): Milton, what an imagination!

FATHER: I wish it were a dream. Then I could wake up. We're living in a nightmare.

MOTHER: But I'm grateful, Milton, that you're willing to become a vegetarian. Ellen . . .

FATHER (*interrupting*): I'm not willing! I'll eat peas and salads if that helps Ellen, but I long for a good dish of kalbshaxe!

MOTHER: I know you're making sacrifices because you love Ellen.

FATHER: If only I could be sure that it helps her.

MOTHER: I think it does. She's very excited about learning all there is to know about lentils. She's studying how to grow them, and cook them, and even their history.

FATHER: Yes, but we're the ones who eat most of her dishes, and later we pass gas . . . oh yes, very gently, so as not to be embarrassed. She's satisfied with the aesthetics.

MOTHER: No, Milton. I've been watching her. She really is eating more.

FATHER: Yes, but I think she's taking laxatives. I found a bottle in the bathroom.

MOTHER: It wasn't the one that the doctor prescribed for you?

FATHER: I know my own medication.

MOTHER: Then I'll throw it away. I'm weighing her every Saturday, and she gained weight this last month.

FATHER: Do you notice what's happening to us?

MOTHER: What do you mean?

FATHER: We talk only about Ellen, even when she isn't here.

MOTHER: Let's change the subject. Let's start dinner.

FATHER: Fine. What's the gourmet pea dish we have tonight?

MOTHER: Don't laugh. I cooked dinner tonight. I thought maybe that would help me understand Ellen better.

FATHER: You're fined 50 marks.

MOTHER: Why?

FATHER: You mentioned Ellen.

MOTHER: You're right. I'm sorry. I prepared stuffed tomatoes and brown rice. (*Walks toward kitchen.*)

FATHER: Stuffed with mincemeat?

MOTHER: Poor Milton. No, stuffed with chick peas, but it's very tasty. (*Goes into kitchen and returns almost immediately with a covered dish on a tray.*) Actually it's a very complicated kind of cooking. I started yesterday.

FATHER: Yesterday? For a pot of lentils?

MOTHER (*serves the food as she talks*): Well, you wash the beans, soak them in cold water overnight, rinse them, boil and rinse them again, and then you cook them for an hour and a half.

FATHER: I calculate about four hours of labor just to have basic chick peas.

MOTHER: Then I took tomatoes, fried onions and garlic, mixed in the chick peas, mashed the whole concoction, and added basil, sea salt, black pepper, and lemon juice. I put it in the oven for forty minutes and here you are: tomatoes stuffed with chick peas.

FATHER: What about the brown rice?

MOTHER: Now you want to know how to fix rice?

FATHER: No, please, no. I was distracted. I was thinking . . .

MOTHER: What?

FATHER: Ellen isn't here today. Why don't we eat like normal people?

MOTHER: She'd find out.

FATHER: How?

MOTHER: I don't know. She'd ask Mary, go smell the kitchen, look for clues in the garbage. I don't know how, but she would.

FATHER: Martha, I feel like a prisoner.

MOTHER: What do you mean?

FATHER: It's Ellen. She's taken over. Our lives are regulated by her needs.

MOTHER: She's sick.

FATHER: But we're not! Why are we eating what she says?

MOTHER: I don't know, Milton. I really don't. I'm so worried about her. I watch her wasting away, and I feel so helpless.

FATHER: I'm not blaming you. You're a mother. I'm surprised at the way *I* have changed—and I suppose you're also becoming an expert on the history of the bean.

MOTHER: Well, the Greeks and Romans used them for casting votes, white ones for pro and colored ones for . . .

FATHER: No, please! It was supposed to be a joke. (*They begin to eat in silence.*)

(*Ellen, the judge, and the parents move to their previous positions, Ellen and her parents again in the docks.*)

JUDGE: This is very damaging evidence. Can you defend yourself?

ELLEN: I didn't know they felt that way.

JUDGE: That is no defense in a court of law.

MOTHER: Children never know what parents suffer. They keep looking at us as if we keep growing taller. Isn't that true, Your Honor?

JUDGE: Indeed it (*stops abruptly*) . . . Madam, don't do that again! You cannot support the accused. This material is presented as evidence against her.

FATHER: I beg the court's indulgence for my wife's behavior. Actually, Your Honor, that's my colleague's style of challenging the defense—turning the other cheek, expressing love when she treats us unfairly. It's a very effective instrument in a woman's hands, Your Honor.

JUDGE: I see. In that case, I'll accept your line of attack. (*To Ellen*) Can you offer anything in your defense?

ELLEN (*stands*): You were eating alone?

FATHER: Yes.

ELLEN: Where was your daughter?

FATHER: She was visiting a friend.

ELLEN: You're certain she was not at home?

MOTHER: You know that you went—

ELLEN: Answer my question! Was she or wasn't she at home?

MOTHER: She was not.

ELLEN: Then why were you feeding her ghost? Why were you acting as if she were there?

FATHER: Because we're concerned about you!

MOTHER: You're so thin.

ELLEN: Your Honor, the accused was exactly ten kilometers from the scene of the crime. She could not have exerted even minimal control over her parents' behavior. The prosecution is using psychological double talk, assigning responsibility to the accused for acts she could not possibly have committed!

MOTHER: But you used your diary before, and we accepted your feelings as evidence against us.

ELLEN: I don't have to play by your rules any more. We're in a court of law. Aren't we, Your Honor?

JUDGE: I doubt it very much. You're making mincemeat of two hundred years of legal procedure. I will rule that the parents' evidence be entered in the record: psychological coercion can be exerted by children at a distance of ten kilometers.

ELLEN (*pauses a moment, then rallies*): May I take my turn now, Your Honor?

JUDGE: Proceed.

(*Lights to black*)

Scene 5

(*There is now a large mirror at center stage. Ellen is writing in her diary; the parents and the judge sit in the background.*)

ELLEN: *I am surrounded by enemies. Wherever I turn, a man stands there with a drawn sword. As on the stage, the unhappy one rushes toward the exit. Stop. An armed man confronts him. He rushes to a second, a third exit . . . all in vain. He's surrounded. He can no longer get out. He collapses in despair. So it is with me. I am in prison, and cannot get out.* (*She stands and studies herself in the large mirror.*) You're imprisoned in your body, Ellen, and you're concerned with external jailers. But they watch me like hawks. How am I holding my fork? Am I dawdling over my food, or am I taking a morsel straight from the plate to my mouth? Am I chewing? And most important, am I swallowing? Their surveillance is pathetic! (*She looks in the mirror, acting out what she describes.*) The vacant glance, as if they're thinking of something else. Catching me out of the corner of their eyes. The 180-degree turn—the look that starts far away and moves casually till it reaches me, and then rushes past, careful not to touch me. The fast, furtive look, frightened, gazelle-like. And the changes in their mood when I eat! Every swallow wins a smile from my mother, and Papa's face relaxes. I feel their heavy gratitude for this act of submission—and I feel guilty. I know—and they don't—that I'll vomit it up in an hour. (*Studies herself again in the mirror.*) I watch them watching me, I watch myself being watched, and I try to achieve a movement that nobody sees. Like this. (*Looks in the mirror, glancing from one side to the other, then puts a fork quickly in her mouth.*) Did they see me? Was I quick enough? Did I manage to take a bite without their thanks? Could they know if the fork had food on it or was empty? I have to be fast. I have to beat them at this game of fattening your daughter! (*She rehearses various gestures— cutting meat, eating quickly, chewing slowly and swallowing. She pretends to put food in her mouth and spit it into a napkin.*) I'll imitate the magician. Nothing in my left hand, nothing in my right. I'll create a diversion, and move so fast they won't know whether I eat or not. The mouth must be faster than the eye—yes, I think I can do it. They will not control my body; it's the only thing that is mine. (*She goes to a scale and weighs herself, then returns to the table and picks up two rocks. She hides them in her pockets, then weighs herself again.*) I've got to find heavier stones.

JUDGE: The attorney for the prosecution will approach the bench. (*Ellen crosses to him.*) Are you sure this is evidence against your parents?

ELLEN: Yes, Your Honor.

JUDGE: It can be used against you as well. But all right, go ahead. Please follow procedures. (*He gestures to the parents, who take their places in the dock.*)

ELLEN (*pacing to and fro*): At this stage in my life, my language was full of holes. I had no words for direct disagreement. My father kept them under lock and key. And my mother took away all words for the middle range of distance. I could only be very close or not close at all. They even punched holes in my verbs. I did the only thing I could do to survive, Your Honor. I became devious. I lied. I crossed my fingers when I promised something, so that I wasn't really committed.

MOTHER: May we speak to that, Your Honor?

JUDGE: Yes. Please begin.

MOTHER: The prosecution is presenting us with an old and tired sophism: I am telling you that I am a liar; therefore, I am sincere. Can we accept her evidence? I will demonstrate that she is telling the truth—she is indeed a liar. Ellen, did you go to Sicily at the age of twenty-one?

ELLEN: You know I did.

MOTHER: And before that, you visited your brother in America?

ELLEN: Yes. What is the relevance of this line of—

MOTHER: When you used to go to the mountains for the summer, who packed your suitcase?

ELLEN: You used to help me. You taught me how to do it, but in the end, you only helped me.

MOTHER: Do you have many friends?

ELLEN: Your Honor, I don't see where the prosecution is going.

JUDGE: Neither do I. But you could accommodate a little. It would make things easier. Could you?

ELLEN: All right. But I'll do it for you, not for her.

JUDGE: Thank you. Proceed, Madam.

MOTHER: How many friends?

ELLEN: You know—Frieda, Sara, Martha.

MOTHER: How often do you visit them?

ELLEN: Well, not very often.

MOTHER: Would you say you go to visit once a week? Once a month? Once a year?

ELLEN: Once a month, I suppose.

MOTHER: And does your mother push you to go more often?

ELLEN: You *nag!* "Why don't you call Frieda?" "I saw Martha today; she said she misses you." Always telling me what to do. Always trying to control me!

MOTHER: The witness has stated quite clearly that her mother encourages her to get away from home, even to the point of pushing her out. Just the opposite of her testimony. Clearly the witness told the truth—she *is* a liar, Your Honor. The defense rests.

ELLEN: You twisted my words! That's what you always do! (*She begins to cry.*) In the end you always get the upper hand, even when you're wrong!

FATHER: Mother didn't want to hurt you, Ellen.

MOTHER: I'm sorry, dear. Please—

JUDGE: Order! Order in the court! I will not accept this level of proximity. Closeness distorts your perspective; truth requires distance. That's why Justice is blind, so that she can see without distortion. Whose turn is it now?

FATHER: Our turn.

JUDGE: All right. Proceed.

(*Lights to black*)

Scene 6

(Ellen and Father sit at the table. The judge and Mother are in the background.)

FATHER: All right, Ellen. We've decided to accept your request. You may eat alone, and that way you can be sure that nobody is looking at what you eat. But we're concerned about you. We see you wasting away, and we long to help you. Please don't tie our hands.

ELLEN: You know I don't want to upset you. But I feel possessed. My world is becoming narrower. My work at the Children's Home used to give me a sense of purpose, but now—I don't know. I love the children. Their eyes don't see my ugliness. But the other day I was with Ernst. He's ten years old, very bright and very sad. Suddenly I had an urge to eat, and I ran. I ran and ran, and behind me, within me, surrounding me, was a vision of a loaf of bread, just taken from the oven, warm to the touch. I walked fifteen kilometers to put distance between the temptation and myself, but it was with me all the time!

FATHER: Why couldn't you eat just a little bit? Enough to satisfy your palate, control your hunger? When you were little you had such an exquisite sense of discipline. You wanted to be first in your class, and you were. When you took up horseback riding, nobody could compete with you. You could use that discipline to control your obsession.

ELLEN: You don't understand. That *is* what I'm doing. I hate fat. I hate ugliness—superfluous eating when people are poor. I want the leanness of an ascetic life. And I use my will power in pursuit of that life!

FATHER: I don't understand what you're talking about. It must be clear even to you that it's nonsense. You're killing your mother. She's becoming depressed, watching you waste away. Our life has become a battleground. We argue all the time about what we should do with you. How to help you against yourself—since you *are* against yourself. And you defeat us every time.

ELLEN: Papa, I don't want to hurt you or Mama. Tell me what to do!

FATHER: Mama creeps around the house like a ghost. You know how proud she used to be of your companionship—how close you two were, how she could anticipate your every wish. Now she feels guilty. She blames herself for your condition. She says maybe we have controlled your life too much. That maybe we should have encouraged your engagement to Michael.

ELLEN: No. You were right. Just as you were about Georges. I shouldn't try to make decisions. I could pursue a dream, and find myself in a nightmare. You only want what's best . . .

FATHER: It was your mother's doing. She's been upset since you left for the university—quiet, didn't talk much with me. And when she did talk it was about you, or Sam, or David. You know, Sam is doing very well in America. He's like a gentile. No anxieties, no doubts, no guilt.

ELLEN: What about David?

FATHER: He writes to Mama. I don't know about him. He's not like my family. He's concerned with small things: bowel movements, migraines. He's anxious without greatness.

ELLEN: You always said I'm like you when you were young.

FATHER: That was before. You've changed. And we've changed (*his voice grows tense*). We revolve around you. You prepare dishes you insist we must eat, but you don't even taste them. Food, calories, diets; peas, celery, and carrots; lean milk and lean cheese; laxatives and thyroid pills: I'm bored with following you and Mother and accepting your tyranny! You can eat alone now if you want to. But you can't control my eating! From now on if you prepare food and bring it to our table, I'll throw it away! Do you understand?

ELLEN: Papa, I don't want to impose on you. Things will be better—you'll see.

(*Ellen sits on Father's lap, smiling tenderly. Father puts his arm around her, then pushes her off, stands up, and addresses himself to the judge. The others resume trial positions.*)

FATHER: There was no doubt, Your Honor, that she was lying. We know all her tricks. But we don't know what to do! We're like deep sea divers who have no clue where the surface is. Sometimes I say to Martha, "This way. Clearly, this must be the way." And she says, "No, no. This must be the deep part. Let's try that way." We argue, and we each insist we know the way out, but we know that we are lying to ourselves. We're in despair!

JUDGE: Bravo, Counselor! That was an impassioned speech. This kind of appeal will certainly impress the jury. Is the defense ready?

ELLEN: Yes, Your Honor, but it will not be helpful. I don't want their control, but I can't move without them. I'm their puppet. I move my arms as if my parents are pulling the strings (*makes a movement like a marionette*). If I'm eating and they don't watch me, I feel as if somebody mislaid the script. I stop again until they notice. We prompt each other. We feed each other lines. And we are so predictable.

JUDGE: Your point is too subjective. Pathos works better in the hands of the prosecution. But who knows? Do you want to add something, Madam? Something short?

MOTHER: All right. (*She sighs audibly.*)

JUDGE: We're at the midpoint in the trial, but we're still at the beginning. I don't know who to judge any more. Who is on trial? Who is the accuser? I feel I'm in quicksand! We will follow proper procedures! I will accept no more of this sentimental babble. There will be respect for the bench. Is that clear?

ELLEN
AND PARENTS: Yes, Your Honor.

JUDGE: Proceed.

(*Lights to black*)

Scene 7

(*Ellen, Father, and Mother are seated at the table, with the judge in the background. Diet books, charts, large and small scales, and exercise equipment clutter the room. Dishes and cups are piled high on the table.*)

FATHER: That does it. You've been lying to us, to the doctor, and to yourself. For six months we've watched you wasting away, and nobody said a thing. But I know you've got on layers of clothing so no one will see how thin you are. I see you trembling when it isn't cold out. You've stopped . . . er . . . your monthlies, and you're abusing your body with laxatives. From now on you'll eat with us again, and YOU WILL EAT!

MOTHER (*putting her hand on Father's arm to calm him*): Enough, Papa. I think Ellen understands.

ELLEN (*to Mother*): But when I look at myself in the mirror, I see I'm still fat (*blows her cheeks out*).

FATHER: Then I'll cover all the mirrors in the house. We'll be your mirrors. *We'll* tell you how you look, how you feel, and when you're hungry!

ELLEN (*with equal intensity*): I'm twenty-eight years old! I work, I go to classes, I've traveled all over Europe! (*She pinches the skin on her hands.*) And I love Karl, and I want to marry him! You haven't experienced all that for me. *I* have!

MOTHER: Ellen, we're not talking about experience or independence. We're talking about survival. Papa could make a list of his experiences twice as long as yours, but you've taken *our* independence away! We had to eat your gourmet dishes that you wouldn't touch. Whose body were we? We couldn't take vacations because you were afraid of being alone. Whose body were we then? You insisted that I read your diet books, and we all became vegetarians. Who did your skin cover then?

FATHER: Enough, Mama. Please serve dinner.

(*Mother serves the food, carefully giving Ellen the same amounts that she gives Father. They all begin to eat. The parents look constantly at Ellen, who is dawdling over her food, using the fork to separate all the ingredients into separate piles on the plate. Mother looks at Father, indicating that he should not interfere. At that moment Ellen shoves half her food into the handbag in her lap, then picks up a morsel and chews obviously. She smiles at Mother, who is watching her again.*)

ELLEN: You're right. I'm behaving like a spoiled child. I know that all you want is to see me well again—and so does Karl. We went hiking last weekend. It's absolutely the right time to enjoy the autumn. Every tree is a kaleidoscope of colors. You have to catch Nature in a moment of distraction, when she doesn't realize that she's dying. She lies beautifully then, promising . . . But next week the trees will be bare.

MOTHER (*looking at Ellen's plate*): Please, Ellen, eat a little bit more. We're almost finished and you're still dawdling.

ELLEN: But, Mama, I've eaten almost half what you gave me. Much more than I eat when I'm alone. And you gave me a portion larger than Papa's and you know I don't like gravy. Ugh! The food is *covered* with gravy!

MOTHER (*passing the bread*): Well, mop up the gravy with the bread, and then you can eat the rest of the food.

FATHER: We're entering her little games again, Martha. Don't you see what she's doing to you?

MOTHER: I don't mind it. At least she's eating. When you demand she feels attacked—and she's right. She's not a child any more, Milton.

FATHER: So now she's not eating because of me! I'm harsh with her!

MOTHER: I didn't say that.

FATHER: No, but you implied it.

ELLEN: Please don't argue about me!

FATHER: She's always manipulated you. If you could only have been more firm with her—

MOTHER: Now, Milton. Ellen has promised that she'll eat.

FATHER: She has promised so many times. Why do you believe her? How is it that she's managed to make you her puppet? She pulls the strings in such a devious way that *she* seems to be manipulated.

MOTHER: What's wrong with loving your own child, and protecting her when she's sick?

FATHER: Because it's—look at what's happening to us. We never used to argue!

ELLEN: Stop it! (*She rises in agitation.*) Please stop it!

(*Her handbag falls, spilling its contents on the floor. Father and Mother look with horror at the food, then Father scoops up the bag and throws its contents on the table. He picks up the objects, identifying them one by one.*)

FATHER: An old baked potato. Crumbled cookies. An apple. A stale piece of bread. Thyroid pills. Laxatives. More pills. Suppositories. A bottle (*reading label*), "Somnifem." Gravy from today's dinner (*wipes his hands on a napkin*). A piece of meat. Where does your skin end, Ellen? Where are the walls of your stomach? (*Turns the purse upside down and shakes it.*) What kind of private hell have you made for us?

(*Ellen hangs her head, weeping silently.*)

JUDGE: We're back at the beginning. You refuse to respect the forms of the law. The prosecution defends the accused; the defense testifies against itself. How can I distinguish the opponents if you keep changing sides? How can I find the guilty party? Court will recess for fifteen minutes. (*He looks savagely at the audience.*) The jury will return in exactly fifteen minutes. Is that clear?

(*Curtain*)

Act 2, Scene 1

(*As in the previous act, the stage has a table and two chairs, but it is a slightly different room. The room is clean, and the mood at the beginning of the first scene is calm and companionable. The judge, Father, Mother, Ellen, and Karl enter, carrying their chairs. The judge sits in his large chair in the middle of the stage. Father and Mother sit together on one side, facing Ellen and Karl.*)

JUDGE (*to Karl*): What are you doing here?

KARL: Ellen told me I should come.

JUDGE: Only the participants in the trial may sit here. If you're a member of the jury, you must sit with them. (*Embarrassed, Karl gets up and moves to the front of the stage, looking for a way to descend to the audience.*)

ELLEN: But Your Honor, he's my husband!

JUDGE: You don't see my wife sitting with me, do you?

MOTHER: But he's part of the trial, Your Honor.

JUDGE: Another one of your tricky maneuvers, Counselor?

MOTHER: No, Your Honor. I'm afraid he may become an accessory to Ellen's murder.

ELLEN (*annoyed*): How can you say that? You don't know anything about our relationship.

MOTHER: That's precisely the point. Why don't I know?

ELLEN: Because I don't tell you, that's why.

MOTHER: You hardly write to us. You only came to visit us twice in the past six months.

ELLEN: Yes, but I stayed a week each time.

MOTHER: Yes, but he didn't come. And you're not confiding in me any more. He's poisoning our relationship, trying to create distance between us.

FATHER: But, Martha, he's her husband.

MOTHER: Don't you take his side! Don't you see what he's doing?

FATHER: Yes, helping her grow up.

MOTHER: You're making me feel foolish again, as if it was all my fault. What about you? What about your control and your doting—

ELLEN: Please! Please! I don't live at home any more.

KARL (*to Judge*): It's all nonsense, the notion of this trial. We have problems like all families, and we'll solve them alone.

JUDGE: Not all families have an attempted murder.

FATHER: You can't know, Your Honor. You only know the ones that come to trial.

KARL (*to Ellen*): Let's stop this charade.

MOTHER (*to Judge*): Can they do that, Your Honor? Can they just not come?

JUDGE: No, Madam. I can always subpoena them. But I'm curious. What is your accusation?

MOTHER: I charge my son-in-law with alienation of my daughter's affection.

JUDGE: But that's irrelevant in a murder trial.

MOTHER: Not really, Your Honor, because if she moves away from us we can't save her.

FATHER: You're losing your sanity, Martha!

ELLEN: But Your Honor, I don't have a problem any more.

FATHER: Can you prove that?

KARL (*gets up; Ellen follows him, putting her arms around him and looking up at him*): Of course we can. But I don't want to. We don't have to prove anything.

JUDGE: I'm afraid you do. (*In a more familiar tone, he explains to Karl*). You see, the law protects your rights. Your home is your castle. But once you put down the drawbridge and let us in, you must follow procedures.

KARL: What do we have to do?

ELLEN: We have to present evidence on our behalf. I know the form. Just follow me.

JUDGE: Is the defense ready? (*Ellen nods.*) Proceed, then.

(*The judge and parents move to the background. Ellen brings two chairs to the table, which is set for breakfast. She takes a piece of toast from the grill, butters it, and pours herself a cup of coffee. Karl takes his chair to the table and joins her, yawning.*)

ELLEN: Good morning, dearest! Coffee? (*He nods. She pours him coffee and he begins to drink. She eats the toast deliberately, chewing slowly and with enjoyment.*) Look, the Dybbuk has gone! Hooray for the exorcist!

KARL: It was your doing, not mine. Pass me the toast? (*She butters a piece for him.*)

ELLEN: It was your respecting my meanderings. I feel safe with you.

KARL (*eating*): I try to be where you need me—the right place at the right time.

ELLEN: That's promising a lot.

KARL: Will you help me?

ELLEN: Wait a minute. I thought you were the helper.

KARL: Yes, but can't you help the helper once in a while?

ELLEN: You're cheating again! Here I was so certain, and you pulled the rug out from under me.

KARL: It still leaves you firm floor. What more do you want?

ELLEN: I want all of you, every bit of you.

KARL: You have me. How can you doubt it? You're brilliant and beautiful.

ELLEN: Really? Beautiful?

KARL: Beautiful as the Queen of Sheba.

ELLEN: And is my body thin and voluptuous?

KARL (*gets up, picks her up from her chair and moves his hands, delineating her body*): Mmmm (*touching her hips with his hands*), it could be rounder here and there.

ELLEN: You see? You don't like me.

KARL: I love you. I want more of you.

ELLEN: Cheater! You want to fatten me up.

KARL (*kisses her, then holds her chin, looking at her face*): I want to drink from you and be drunk all my life.

ELLEN: Now I know why you married me. You're a secret alcoholic.

KARL (*leads her to his chair and sits her on his lap*): Finally discovered! I won't have to hide it any more. By the way, I have a surprise for you.

ELLEN: A present?

KARL: No, not really. Guess again.

ELLEN: I give up.

KARL: You didn't even try. All right, I bought tickets for the concert Sunday night. We could go out for dinner first. I'm sure you'll love it. It's the *St. Matthew Passion,* played on original instruments.

ELLEN: Mmmm, I don't know.

KARL: But you always seem to search for the original forms. I was so sure you'd like it—

ELLEN: Please, Karl, don't read me! You promised not to become my parents.

KARL: You're so sensitive. I thought you'd like it.

ELLEN: That's what I mean. *You* thought *I'd* like it—guessing my thinking.

KARL: Then we won't go.

ELLEN: Now *you* decide that *we* won't go. No, you bought the tickets, we'll go. But please don't do that anymore *(gets up and paces restlessly)*.

KARL: Ellen, please. Give me time. I'll find the right way. Look, I—

ELLEN *(pulls away from Karl, who stops midword; goes to the table, where there is a plate of fruit)*: I think I'll have an apple. No. A peach. *(She turns away from Karl and bites into it.)*

(Karl springs up and angrily sweeps the plate off the table; it falls, scattering the fruit. Father, in the background, jumps to his feet. Mother grabs his arm.)

KARL: Don't you do that! *(Ellen whirls toward him, surprised and frightened.)* Don't escape from me into your world of apples and peaches! I wanted to please you, all right? All right? *(He speaks more gently.)* Clearly, I was wrong. I don't know how to do it. But I'm trying! And what do you do? You're considering the transcendent virtues of peaches and apples!

ELLEN *(comes to Karl, a placating smile on her face. She gives him the peach. He takes it, not knowing what to do with it.)* I'm sorry, Karl, I truly am. But I'm also glad. It's reassuring to know you'll protect me from my obsessions.

FATHER *(springs from his chair and goes to Karl)*: It's a trap! Don't step in it! It's quicksand. I was up to my neck in it!

(Karl and Ellen look at him in surprise. The judge moves his chair forward, to the trial position. The others follow.)

JUDGE *(to Father)*: Do you wish to cross-examine?

KARL: Your Honor, I don't believe that this trial should continue. Things have changed.

JUDGE: Not in a legal sense. The accusation still stands.

MOTHER (*looking at Father*): May the prosecution take time for a conference?

JUDGE: By all means.

MOTHER: Milton, can we trust Karl?

FATHER: He's my nephew. I think we can trust him.

MOTHER: But look how angry he got! And only because she selected a peach instead of an apple!

FATHER: There you go, protecting her again. She's married to him. She's his responsibility, not ours.

MOTHER: I could never forgive myself if anything happened to her.

FATHER: Martha, please. Let her go. We can take a vacation from being parents.

(*As they talk, he begins automatically to pick up the fruit from the floor. Mother picks up the plate. As they put the things on the table, they look at each other and laugh.*)

MOTHER (*to Karl*): Will you call me if Ellen needs me?

JUDGE: Does the prosecution wish to reconsider their plea?

FATHER: May we have a minute more, Your Honor?

JUDGE (*with a gesture of resignation*): Go ahead.

MOTHER: Karl?

KARL: Yes?

MOTHER: Will you?

KARL: You can talk with Ellen directly. I'm not her voice.

MOTHER: She will not call me. I know her.

ELLEN: You don't know me, Mother. You only know your daughter.

MOTHER: You *are* my daughter.

KARL: She's also my wife.

ELLEN (*looks at Mother, then at Karl*): Is this what I am?

MOTHER: You know she was my daughter before she became your wife.

JUDGE: Has the prosecution reached an agreement?

FATHER: Just a minute, Your Honor. Martha, we must stop the trial. Ellen is not our responsibility any more.

MOTHER: How can you say that? She'll always be our responsibility. You will write to me, Ellen? Will you come to visit us?

ELLEN: Of course, Mother. (*She looks at Karl, who makes a gesture of agreement.*) You and Father can always come to visit us too.

JUDGE: Well?

FATHER: Your Honor, we wish to withdraw our plea and end the trial.

JUDGE (*to Ellen*): There is still the case of grand larceny against your parents.

ELLEN: What do you think, Karl? Should I stop accusing them? They made me what I am.

FATHER: That's not so bad.

KARL: I think you should stop the trial. We're two now. Together we can select new words.

ELLEN: I think you're right. (*To judge*) I want to stop the trial of my parents.

JUDGE (*to Karl*): Can I perchance be of service to you?

KARL: I don't believe in trials. It's a waste of time and money. Besides, you demand clarity, and I'm always half angry and half guilty.

JUDGE: There is no need to be rude, young man. (*Rises.*) Court adjourned.

(*The parents leave. The judge takes his chair to the corner of the stage and sits there, observing Karl and Ellen.*)

KARL (*gesturing in the direction of the parents' exit*): They'll always be there, ready to be summoned.

ELLEN: I won't call them. But they're old, you know. Now that I'm married, they don't have anybody.

KARL: They have each other, just as we do.

ELLEN: Not in the same way. They're locked in old routines. It's strange, you know. I always thought I was dependent on them, and now I realize that without me their life loses meaning.

KARL: Of course. But if you give them time, they'll invent new games.

ELLEN: We can invent new things too. Will you help me?

KARL: Sure. In what way?

ELLEN: Let's have a child.

KARL (*surprised*): To give meaning to your parents' lives?

ELLEN: No, silly. To celebrate. To celebrate the me that likes myself because you like me.

KARL: Do you want a boy or a girl?

ELLEN: Do you have a way of choosing?

KARL: You order and I'll package it—him or her—for you.

ELLEN (*sitting on his lap*): I want a little girl.

(*They kiss. Alarmed, the judge coughs to make his presence known. Ellen and Karl jump to their feet.*)

KARL: Who's there?

JUDGE: I'm sorry. I thought you knew I was here.

KARL: Why? What are you doing here? The trial is over. You're trespassing.

JUDGE: I wish that were true.

ELLEN: What do you mean?

JUDGE: The trial is not over.

KARL: We dismissed you.

JUDGE: But I cannot leave.

ELLEN: But you must!

JUDGE: I'm sorry. One of the problems of justice is its cumbersome machinery. After you switch it off it continues running for a while, just by inertia, until it stops on its own.

KARL: How long can it last?

JUDGE: Not long. Sometimes a couple of years. Sometimes longer. But if you accept my presence, I promise to be discreet. (*He takes off his robe. He's wearing a checked sports shirt and slacks.*)

ELLEN: What will you be doing?

JUDGE: I'll keep you under surveillance.

ELLEN: Why?

JUDGE: Once you find a suspect, you keep her under surveillance.

KARL: That's ridiculous. She's not guilty of anything.

JUDGE: Most people are. You're a suspect too.

KARL: Me? What did I do?

JUDGE: You have a violent temper; you made fraudulent promises—telling Ellen that you could protect her against herself; and now you are offering her a child with a specific gender, a promise you know you can't make good on.

KARL: That's cheating! You observe my behavior, you describe it, and then you accuse me of my own behavior!

JUDGE: Certainly.

KARL: But by that method everybody can become a suspect.

JUDGE: That's true.

KARL: Why?

JUDGE: There is no alternative.

ELLEN: Can we do anything to get rid of you?

JUDGE: If you can accept my presence, I become almost invisible.

Most people grow accustomed to surveillance. After all, it starts
at home, very early.

KARL: Can we make a deal?

JUDGE: We're always making them.

KARL: First, you don't tell her parents what happens between us.
Second, you don't enter our bedroom.

JUDGE: No to the first, yes to the second.

KARL: It's a deal. (*Shakes judge's hand and turns to Ellen.*) Let's go to
the bedroom.

(*They leave. The judge remains on stage, at a loss.*)

(*Lights to black*)

Scene 2

(*The judge sits unobtrusively in a corner of the stage. Ellen walks
back and forth, holding a blanket in her arms cradled like a baby. Rocking
it back and forth, she sings a lullaby, then begins talking in a dreamlike
mood.*)

ELLEN: My poor little girl . . . I lost her. I pushed her out. It was
midday in Spring. We stopped near the brook. Karl put the
bottle of wine in the water. He ate a sandwich of cheese and
lettuce. I ate seven apples, or was it fourteen? Never mind. The
clouds had the shape of children's toys—elephants, a seesaw, a
very large whale, a teddy bear, a baby carriage, a pain—an intense pain in the center of my being. I hear a baby cry. Hold
on! The laxatives? Yesterday I took seven, but I will hold on.
I will not defecate my little girl. The clouds . . . "Look, Karl," I
said, "look at this cloud—the one like a giant birthday cake." I
held on. We were in the middle of Spring, ten kilometers from
town. We walked slowly. A pain in my center . . . but I didn't
vomit. I held on to my girl step after step, thinking: How many
laxatives did I have last night? Seven? No, more than that. But
I will not expel my little girl. I will hold on. I will hold on.
"Breathe deeply," the doctor said, "It won't hurt. I will finish
soon. Just scraping." Now I have excreted from all my ori-
fices—I'm empty. "Karl," I said, "look at this cloud." "What
cloud?" he said. "Never mind. It's already changed shape."

JUDGE (*approaching Ellen*): I'm sorry. I'm very sorry.

ELLEN: It's not your function to be sorry. You're here only to prove my guilt.

JUDGE: But that's exactly the issue. You're not guilty.

ELLEN: Who is?

JUDGE: Nobody is.

ELLEN: It was my body, wasn't it?

JUDGE: Didn't you conceive with the collaboration of your husband?

ELLEN: Yes, but it was my body.

JUDGE: Why did your husband take you walking so far in your condition? Why didn't he protect you as he promised?

ELLEN: I know what you're doing. You want to put the blame on Karl. But the man only plants the seed. The responsibility is the woman's alone.

JUDGE: I only want to point out that accidents happen.

ELLEN: That wasn't an accident. It was murder.

JUDGE: No jury of your peers would say so.

ELLEN: *I* say so. My body did it. It has always been against me. It insists that I can't control it. But I will! (*Ellen takes off her dress, oblivious to the judge, who goes back to his chair. She is dressed in a black leotard. Looking at herself in the mirror, she takes a crayon and draws a pear on her abdomen. On her breasts she draws apples. Then she begins to do bending exercises, counting aloud from the number sixty.*) Sixty-one, sixty-two, sixty-three ... yes, seventy. A multiple of seven. (*Studying her abdomen.*) It was my body. It does what I tell it. If I say bend, it bends. If I say eat, it will eat. It doesn't obey anybody but me ... what now? Ah, the feast.

(*She looks around the room, finds a bowl and puts it on the table. She breaks eggs into the bowl, cracking each with one hand, slowly and ritualistically. She counts aloud, "1, 2, 3, 4, 5, 6, 7," then puts seven spoonfuls of sugar in the bowl, moving quickly, in contrast to the slowness of the egg cracking. She beats the eggs, then takes seven tomatoes and seven apples out of a box, lining them up on the table. When she has finished she looks around, finds a bottle of pills, and carefully counts out seven.*)

ELLEN: The laxatives. Exactly seven, like the eggs, sugar, apples, and tomatoes. They have to cancel out each other. (*Looking at her abdomen.*) It is *my* body! (*She takes the blanket in her arms and begins to rock it back and forth, singing a lullaby.*)

(*Lights to black*)

Scene 3

(The office of an analyst. Ellen is lying on the couch. The analyst is seated on a chair behind her. The judge sits in the corner of the stage.)

ELLEN: *I think only about my body, my eating, my laxatives. It was easier before, when everything was grey around me, when I wanted nothing but to be sick and lie in bed. Now I like to be healthy but I don't want to pay the price for it.*

ANALYST: M-hm.

ELLEN: *As soon as I feel a pressure at my waist my spirit sinks, and I get a depression so severe, as if it were a question of goodness knows what tragic affair. On the other hand, if I have a good bowel movement there is a kind of calm.*

ANALYST: M-hm.

ELLEN: *I don't think that the dread of becoming fat is the real obsessive neurosis (turns around and looks at the analyst), but the constant desire for food. The pleasure of eating must have been the primary thing. Dread of becoming fat served as a brake, don't you think? (Lies down again.)*

ANALYST: M-hm.

ELLEN: *Anyway, the picture has shifted. A year ago, I looked forward to hunger and then I ate with appetite, and then I took a laxative so that I shouldn't put on fat. Now, in spite of my hunger, every meal is a torment. (Her voice grows dull and automatic, as if she is repeating something she has said many times before.) I'm constantly accompanied by feelings of dread. I feel them like something physical, an ache in my heart. It drives all other thoughts out of my head. Even when I'm full, I'm afraid of the coming hour in which hunger will start again. When I'm hungry I can no longer see anything clear. (She turns to the doctor, speaks in her normal voice.)* Where does this unrest come from, Doctor? Why do I think I can dull it only with food? You might say, "Eat the bread. Then you will have peace." But no. When I've eaten it I'm unhappier than ever. Then I sit and see constantly before me the bread I've eaten. I feel my stomach and keep thinking "Now you will get fat."

ANALYST: *You attempt to satisfy two things while eating: hunger and love. Hunger gets satisfied; love does not. There remains the great unfilled hole.*

ELLEN: Let me sit on your lap and put my head on your shoulder. *(She does this.)* Please call me "Ellen, my child."

JUDGE (*beckoning to Ellen*): Psst! (*Ellen goes to him.*) Are you having an affair with him?

ELLEN: Certainly not.

JUDGE: Why do you sit in his lap?

ELLEN: Oh, that's called transference. I'm reliving my childhood, and I fell in love with him since he's symbolically my father.

JUDGE: Oh. But is that true?

ELLEN: What?

JUDGE: That you equate food with love?

ELLEN: Yes, symbolically it's true.

JUDGE: Isn't it possible that your mother did not love you?

ELLEN: Oh no, she loved me . . . too much.

JUDGE: And your father?

ELLEN: Also. In his own way.

JUDGE: And Karl?

ELLEN: Karl loves me, the way a normal man loves his wife.

JUDGE: So it's all in you.

ELLEN: Yes. I have to solve it—rearrange my old experience inside of me, until I can see today without distortions.

JUDGE: It sounds fishy to me. (*Points to the analyst.*) Do you trust him?

ELLEN: Well, he's brilliant, but at times I think he's too theoretical—but that's called negative transference.

JUDGE (*taking out his notebook*): I'll put him under surveillance.

ELLEN: Why?

JUDGE: I don't know yet.

(*Lights to black*)

Scene 4

(*A hotel room. Ellen and Karl are seated at a table.*)

KARL: The analyst said I shouldn't stay in Switzerland with you. That I should go home. That I interfere with the progress of your therapy.

ELLEN: Please, Karl, don't go! My time is so empty. I need you.

KARL: But the analyst says that I interfere with the transference.

ELLEN: But why can't you stay here and be real, while I work with your distortion inside me? It's frightening to be populated by so many people in my unconscious and to be alone in real life. If you leave, I'll kill myself!

KARL: He says your main goal is subjugating people.

ELLEN: He says . . . he says . . . he says. *I* say I need you. I'm afraid! I see black birds hovering around me.

KARL: Ellen, believe me, I only want to help you. But I don't know the best way. I want to stay here with you, but what if my staying creates problems? He's a doctor. If we don't follow his advice, it's better for you to stop the analysis.

ELLEN: You're right. Everybody's right. (*Her voice grows dull and distant.*) Everybody wants to help me. Father, Mother, you, the doctors. How many doctors? Ten? Twenty? Thirty? (*Her voice changes; she sounds like a ventriloquist's doll.*) Take these pills and your menstruation will return. This one and you'll be able to conceive. You need to take control. Let your unconscious flow. You're overactive. You're depressed. You should work and concentrate on something outside yourself. You should rest and concentrate on your images. We are all helpers. We're helping. We will continue to help (*her voice rises hysterically*).

KARL (*takes her arms and embraces her, trying to calm her*): Ellen, please, take hold of yourself. I won't go. I'll stay with you.

ELLEN (*normal voice*): No, you're right. I have to wrestle with my demons alone. I'll be all right. You can go home.

JUDGE (*joins them at center stage, interrupting*): Forgive me.

KARL: *You* again.

JUDGE: I don't trust her. I smell a rat.

KARL: What do you mean?

JUDGE: The more I think about this case, the less I like it. (*Karl stares at him, nonplussed.*) Too many helpers outside and too many demons inside, and they don't talk to each other.

ELLEN: Could *you* help me?

JUDGE: Helping is not my business! Surveillance is.

ELLEN: So what do you propose to do?

JUDGE: I don't know. But if we could have all your helpers together, perhaps we could allocate responsibility.

ELLEN: Would that help me?

KARL (*disappointed*): That's what you're after? Forget it. It will only create more confusion.

JUDGE: I know. I must be getting old. But you must agree it was a great fantasy. If justice could only have certainty . . . (*He moves slowly back to his chair and sits.*)

KARL (*turns to Ellen*): Are you sure you'll be all right if I go home?

ELLEN: Yes, don't worry. I'll be all right. (*Karl kisses her and leaves the room. Ellen looks after him for a moment, then goes to a shelf with bottles of medicines and looks through them, reading the labels.*) Talk, talk, talk. They spin fantasies. They entertain each other. They argue about my ghosts. Then they leave for their world of purpose and I am alone and useless. (*Picks up a bottle and reads the label.*) "Somnasetine." That would surprise them. I could put the whole menagerie of ghosts to sleep. Fifty-six pills for fifty-six sleeping demons. (*She spills the pills into her hand.*) Yes, that's right. Seven times eight is fifty-six. (*She swallows the pills.*) Tomorrow I will sleep.

(*She goes to the table, pushes the contents to the floor, and lies down on the table. The light fades. She is seen sitting up on the table, and there is a noise of vomiting. The analyst enters in the dim light, and sits behind the table, near her head.*)

ELLEN: It's not fair! (*Her voice grows dull.*) It's *my* body. Last night I wanted to kill myself, but even in dying I fail. I took fifty-six pills of Somnasetine and vomited all of them. Am I condemned to live? (*Speaks like a judge pronouncing sentence.*) "Because you are fat and ugly, we give you fifty years of life."

ANALYST: M-hm.

JUDGE: I knew I couldn't trust her demons.

(*Lights to black*)

Scene 5

(*Ellen and Karl are in a room in a sanatorium. The judge sits in a corner of the stage. The room is clean and bare. They're seated across from each other at a table.*)

KARL: I came as soon as I could. The doctors say you're not safe any more, outside a sanatorium.

ELLEN (*as if talking to herself*): They can control my life, but they will not control my death. That will be my own. There are so many ways of dying. I counted twenty-eight, and I've only used three. I took pills, but I couldn't hold them. I jumped in front of a carriage, but the driver avoided me. I wanted to jump from my analyst's window, and he stopped me. They're condemning me to the life that *they* want. *I feel excluded from real life.*

KARL (*goes to her and takes her hand*): I'm here, Ellen. I'll help you, if you'll only tell me how. Please let me in.

ELLEN (*looking at him for the first time, her voice normal*): No, Karl. My demons are stronger than you. They stuff my ears. I see your lips moving in silence.

KARL: Ellen, your demons must have familiar faces! Don't you recognize me among them?

ELLEN: I only know that inside of me, not outside, there's a struggle between my aspiration to be perfect and my sense of worthlessness, between my thinness and my ugliness.

KARL: *We* are your demons! Our silence is the glass wall you're touching!

ELLEN: Maybe it started that way. But now it's all inside me.

KARL: Don't I exist? Touch me! (*He takes Ellen's hand and directs it toward his face as if guiding a blind person's hand.*) Do you hear my voice? Am I framing your imperfect life? Or am I its builder?

ELLEN: I know you want to carry part of the load. But it's my burden.

KARL: No! It's not only yours. Please, don't make me helpless. Don't escape! Don't run away from me into this useless world of minutiae and food. Let me help you!

ELLEN: Finish your phrase. "Let me help you—empty puppet. Greedy container." (*Distant and automatic*) Every meal is a combination of temptation and anxiety. And the hours in between are empty spaces. I fill them with thoughts of food. (*She looks around and goes to a bowl of fruit. She reaches out, then bends her wrist so she can't touch the food. Looks at Karl.*)

KARL (*angry*): Don't do that! (*Pleading*) Please don't do that. I want to be with you! (*He stands and backs up as he talks.*) But you fill the space between us with words about food. I can't reach you.

ELLEN (*following him, soft and intimate*): I'll tell you about me. All my life I've felt controlled by people—helping people. I used to fight them, but then I realized they were right. Only by listening to them could I know how I felt—cold, hungry, maybe tired. But then the voices began to disagree with each other.

One would say, "You're hungry." "No, you're fat." That's when my demons moved inside.

(*The judge enters, looking official again, wearing his robe and carrying a gavel. He sits facing Karl and Ellen.*)

KARL: We want to resolve this alone.

JUDGE: M-hm.

KARL: This isn't a matter for the courts!

JUDGE: M-hm.

ELLEN: Did my parents send you?

JUDGE: Uh-huh [no].

ELLEN: The doctors?

JUDGE: Uh-huh [no].

ELLEN: If they're not accusing, why are you convening the court?

JUDGE: M-hm.

ELLEN: Why don't you answer?

JUDGE: I've been experimenting with the nuances of M-hm. It has definite possibilities. A certain degree of ambiguity could enhance the court proceedings. It has dignity and power, and the meaning is carried by the accused. Yes, I think the court can use it.

KARL: Why are you starting legal proceedings?

JUDGE: There is a criminal matter unresolved. Ellen has been accused of attempted murder. I simply adjourned the court until more evidence was available.

KARL: Shouldn't Ellen's parents be present? They were the prosecution.

JUDGE: I will call them if necessary. But since there have been five suicide attempts, the court can intervene directly. How do you plead?

ELLEN: Guilty, Your Honor. It's my body. I can dispose of it as I wish.

KARL: Your Honor, Ellen is not competent to conduct a proper defense. I request the court to appoint me her attorney.

JUDGE: You have no legal training.

KARL: No, but we've been married for five years. You know I know her well.

JUDGE: Do you accept him as your attorney?

ELLEN: I don't care. If he wants to defend me he can. But I have to make the decision. Legally, I'm an adult. I own certain properties: a house in Fredrichstrasse, bonds and money in a Swiss bank, a summer cabin near Salzburg, and my body. They are all legally in my name. As long as I pay taxes, I can dispose of them as I like.

KARL: May I begin the defense, Your Honor?

JUDGE: Are you sure you don't want legal advice? Ellen is a most difficult client.

KARL: My wife's reasoning is impaired.

ELLEN: That's not true, Karl. For the first time in my life I know what I want, not what others want me to want.

KARL: Can the defendant's statement be stricken from the record? She cannot testify against herself.

JUDGE: The jury is so advised. Erase your memory (*slaps his head on both sides*).

KARL: Your Honor, the accused labors under the grandiose misconception that she can control her world and that therefore she is solely responsible.

JUDGE: As an adult, she *is* responsible. Are you questioning the legal concept?

KARL: No, Your Honor. I wish to present the extenuating circumstances.

JUDGE: Proceed.

KARL: The defendant was born an infant. She became a toddler, a child, an adolescent, and later an adult. She was helped in this meandering by her parents, brothers, friends, teachers, husband, two analysts, and over a score of members of the medical profession.

JUDGE: Is this your defense? This line of reasoning has no legal validity.

KARL: Your Honor, to state at the age of thirty-three, as the defendant does, that she thinks *her* thoughts, wants *her* wants, makes the *sole* decisions in her life, is sheer folly.

JUDGE: Ah! So you are pleading not guilty by reason of insanity.

KARL: Yes, Your Honor.

ELLEN: That's not so! I am perfectly sane.

JUDGE (*to Karl*): I will accept your plea.

KARL: Ellen, we must understand your illness better. The internist thinks your analyst is not helping you. That he's treating you for the wrong illness. That he's feeding your demons. He would like you to see Dr. Kraepelin, Professor of Psychiatry. What do you think?

ELLEN: I think that at times . . . what do I think? What do I . . . (*dulled voice*). Yes, I think he's right.

(*Lights to black*)

Scene 6

(*A doctor's office in the sanatorium. The judge and Karl are in the background. Multiple diplomas grace the wall. Dr. Kraepelin is seated at a desk, dressed in a white doctor's tunic, with his arms on the desk and his hands clasped. Ellen enters. Dr. Kraepelin rises, shakes her hand formally, touches his heels together, and bows.*)

KRAEPELIN (*formally*): I am Dr. Kraepelin. Please turn around and walk toward the wall. (*She does so.*) Turn around, walk toward me with your eyes closed. Stop. Thank you. Extend your arms and stretch your fingers. (*She follows each of his orders.*) Thank you. (*Makes a gyrating motion with both hands.*) Turn your hands back and forth. Thank you. Extend your right hand and with the index finger touch your nose. Do it again. Thank you. (*Takes a pin from his lapel and pricks Ellen on the forehead. She recoils.*) There is nothing to fear. Stand in front of me. Close your eyes. (*Pricks her forehead with the pin. Ellen winces.*) Did you feel that?

ELLEN: Yes.

KRAEPELIN (*rapidly pricks her face at random, sometimes with the pin, sometimes with his finger. Asks questions staccato, without waiting for answers, so that Ellen, shaking her head yes and no, is always one step behind him.*): Do they feel the same? More? Less? The same? More? Less? Don't guess! Did you feel at all? Tell me if you feel the prick or not. Yes? No? (*Finishing, he puts the pin in his lapel. Ellen opens her eyes.*) Close your eyes. (*Kraepelin takes two steps back, then slowly moves around Ellen until he is in front of her again. He comes closer to examine her eyes, pulling her eyelids down, then touches her throat, feeling the glands with both hands. He moves back to write in his notebook.*) Open your mouth. Stick out your tongue. Move it to the right. To the left. Thank you. Please sit down. (*He sits at his desk and fires off the next questions rapidly.*)

KRAEPELIN: What is your name?

ELLEN: Ellen West.

KRAEPELIN: Age?

ELLEN: Thirty-three.

KRAEPELIN: What day is today?

ELLEN: Tuesday.

KRAEPELIN: Month?

ELLEN: December.

KRAEPELIN: Year?

ELLEN: 1913.

KRAEPELIN: How long have you been here?

ELLEN: Two weeks.

KRAEPELIN: What's my name?

ELLEN: Dr. Kraepelin.

KRAEPELIN: Count to ten. (*Ellen does so.*)

KRAEPELIN: Backward. (*Ellen does so.*)

KRAEPELIN: What is five times seven?

ELLEN: Thirty-five.

KRAEPELIN: Five plus eight plus twenty-two.

ELLEN: Thirty-five.

KRAEPELIN (*as if catching her in an error*): How much?

ELLEN: Thirty-five.

KRAEPELIN: Yes, you're right. (*Writes on chart and reads aloud rapidly.*) Physical appearance: expression depressed, corners of mouth drawn down, emaciated, dry skin, muscle tone increased, salival glands enlarged, thyroid enlarged, mouth dry ... ah, slight hirsutism. Oriented in time and space. Understands questions and answers correctly. (*Looks at Ellen.*) Why are you here?

ELLEN: I want to die.

KRAEPELIN (*sternly*): What else?

ELLEN: I feel a constant wish to eat, and a constant dread of eating.

KRAEPELIN: Constant?

ELLEN: Almost constant. At times I feel better. When my husband—

KRAEPELIN (*interrupting*): When did it start?

ELLEN: My wish to be thin started when I was twenty years old.

KRAEPELIN: How old are you now?

ELLEN: I told you.

KRAEPELIN: Please repeat it.

ELLEN: Thirty-three.

KRAEPELIN: Is there a history of depression in your family?

ELLEN (*automatic tone of voice*): Two of my uncles committed suicide. My father has fears of getting up in the morning. My
brother was hospitalized at the age of seventeen because of ap-
prehension. My grandmother . . .

KRAEPELIN: Maternal or paternal?

ELLEN: Paternal . . . had periods of depression. My aunt had a
nervous breakdown.

KRAEPELIN (*writes, reads aloud*): Family shows depressive tenden-
cies. Do you feel apprehensive?

ELLEN: All the time. I feel a prisoner in a tomb. My demons are
greed and a wish for perfection.

KRAEPELIN: How do they look? What's the color of their eyes?

ELLEN: Who?

KRAEPELIN: Your demons.

ELLEN: Oh, no. I experience them in my internal dialogs.

KRAEPELIN: Do they talk to you? Are they male or female? Harsh
or soft? Commanding or enticing?

ELLEN: No, it's just me talking to myself. Blaming myself for my
greed. For continuing to live in a hell I've constructed.

KRAEPELIN: (*writing and reading*): Delusional ideation. No auditory
or visual hallucinations. Hypochondriacal fears. Obsessive
thoughts about weight. Depressed. (*Thinks, then resumes writing.*)
As a consequence of this mental unrest, patient becomes suicidal. (*Closes the file, studies Ellen, goes to her.*) Mrs. West, you suffer
from melancholia. I will recommend that you stop your analysis and be hospitalized in a different sanatorium. I will talk to
your doctors and prescribe a regimen of life for you. Plenty of
food, plenty of rest, paraldehyde or opium to control your ap-
prehension. Your prognosis is favorable (*turns and goes back to his
desk, begins to write*). (*Ellen hesitates, then understanding that she has
been dismissed, walks to the door.*)

JUDGE: I am impressed, Herr Professor. Just for the record, where
do you teach?

KRAEPELIN: I am Professor of Psychiatry at the University of Heidelberg.

JUDGE: And you are sure of your diagnosis?

KRAEPELIN (*surprised*): I am Professor of Psychiatry at the University of Heidelberg.

JUDGE (*returning to Karl*): Well, I suppose that's an answer.

KARL: I do not question Dr. Kraepelin's competence. But I would like a second opinion.

JUDGE: The court can summon other experts. But you do understand that more opinions will introduce uncertainty?

KARL: Yes, Your Honor.

JUDGE: Proceed, then.

(*Lights to black*)

Scene 7

(*Office setting. At stage right is a platform with a long table and four high-backed chairs facing the audience. Ellen and Karl are seated at stage left. The judge is in the background.*)

ELLEN: I feel like eating a very thick steak, followed by chocolate cake with whipped cream. The condemned should be allowed a last meal.

KARL: Don't think like that. Actually it's a historic moment. You'll be seeing the three most important psychiatrists in Europe.

ELLEN: All except Dr. Freud. I was treated by two of his followers, though. The best that money can buy. The West family always buys quality.

KARL: Don't act cynical. I know you share my excitement and hope.

ELLEN: Yes, it's true. The power of labels. Will they select depression or neurosis, from the white box of words, or schizophrenia, from the black box covered with lead? After the selection, will they paste the label on my forehead? And then will my mind respond accordingly?

KARL: Ellen, I understand that after thirteen years of living with your illness you feel as if you *are* your illness, but—

ELLEN: Is it thirteen years already? Yes, I'm thirty-three. Christ died at thirty-three, and he was also a thin Jew. Do you think Kraepelin knew I was Jewish before he saw me? I've heard he thinks the Jews are dangerous for Germany.

KARL: You know that doctors don't let themselves be guided by their prejudices. They're trained to be objective.

ELLEN: What if they disagree? Each one of them is the best in his field. But what if each one seizes on a different part of me to label? After all, Binswanger disagrees with my analyst's interpretation of my dreams, and Kraepelin recommended that I stop analysis.

KARL: That's why they'll be here together. To explore their disagreements. In the end we'll have the result of their combined wisdom.

ELLEN: Do you really believe in all the things you're saying?

KARL: I believe in science.

ELLEN: Did you know that Inca psychiatrists used to make a hole in their patient's skull, to let the spirits escape? They were the best money could buy at that time.

KARL: There's a great distance between Inca superstition and today's scientific psychiatry.

(*The door opens and Kraepelin, Bleuler, and Binswanger, dressed in white tunics, enter. They sit in the high-backed chairs, so that they look at Karl and Ellen from above. Each carries a placard with his name which he places on the table in front of him. The following scene is played as though in a courtroom, with Ellen and Karl on trial.*)

BINSWANGER (*rises; his manner is formal, pedantic*): Your Honor. Karl and Ellen West. Gentlemen. This meeting is unique in the history of medicine. Mrs. West has attempted suicide five times. Next time she may be successful, unless our opinions demonstrate that psychiatry can help. Our goal, therefore, is not to convince the patient that we can accomplish miracles, but to present our psychiatric point of view about the human being who chose to be Ellen West, and let her choose her destiny. Dr. Bleuler?

(*Bleuler rises. A spotlight picks him out and follows him to center stage, where he talks directly to the audience. The rest of the stage is in darkness.*)

BLEULER: Your Honor, I hope you are acquainted with the basic concepts of my theory of schizophrenia.

JUDGE: You must make it very simple, Professor, so that the jury and I can understand your reasoning. Could you do that, please?

BLEULER: I will try, Your Honor. (*Formally*) In my examination of Frau West, I have found characteristics in her thinking that point clearly to the diagnosis of schizophrenia.

JUDGE: Forgive me, Professor. Can you tell us in simple words what this illness consists of?

BLEULER (*uncomfortable with the interruption*): I was about to, Your Honor. Schizophrenia is a thought disorder. (*Slowly*) It is a disturbance in the way of thinking. Is that sufficiently clear, Your Honor? (*The judge nods and indicates he may continue.*) I have found elements of negativism appearing as early as nine months of age, when Frau West refused to drink milk. The same negativism is manifested today in her suicide attempts and refusal to eat. (*Looks at the judge, who nods again.*) In my examination, I found four predisposing causes of negativism in the patient. (*Holds up one finger.*) Ambitendency, which sets free with every tendency a countertendency. I have seen Frau West extend her arm to pick up a piece of fruit, but toward the end of the movement bend her wrist as far back as it will go, so that her fingers do not reach the fruit. (*Demonstrates the movement, then holds up two fingers.*) Ambivalence, or the tendency to accompany identical ideas with positive and negative feelings at the same time. (*Turns to Ellen*) For instance, Frau West's relation of greed and dread to the bread in the cupboard. (*Holds up three fingers.*) Third, the schizophrenic's splitting of the psyche—for instance, Frau West's dividing herself into the lean, blond aesthete and the fat, ugly, Jewish petit-bourgeoise. And lastly, four (*holds up four fingers*), the imperfect logic of the schizophrenic.

JUDGE: Very impressive, Professor. Thank you. Would it be accurate to say that it's like two people fighting inside of her?

BLEULER (*condescending*): If the court must oversimplify to reach clarity, I would go along.

JUDGE: Thank you, Professor. Kind of you.

(*Bleuler bows to the audience. The stage lights up, and he returns to his chair.*)

JUDGE: Just for the record, Professor, could you state your professional qualifications?

BLEULER: I am Professor of Psychiatry at the University of Zurich.

(*Binswanger points to Kraepelin, who takes center stage.*)

KRAEPELIN: Your Honor. Gentlemen. I disagree with my esteemed colleague. In my opinion, Mrs. West suffers from melancholia. To support the diagnosis of schizophrenia, Professor Bleuler should have documented an instinctive resistance against outer influences. (*Looks at Bleuler and pauses.*) But Mrs. West has always accepted control from outside. Perhaps Professor Bleuler's mistake follows logically from his concentration on thought disturbances, without enough attention to the mood disorders.

JUDGE: What do you mean, Professor?

KRAEPELIN: Disturbances of affect, Your Honor. Melancholia, manic depression, hypomanic states, and so on. Things that have to do in everyday life with being sad or happy.

JUDGE: Thank you, Professor. That was admirable for its clarity and brevity. So it is how you feel—or better, how Mrs. West feels and not how she thinks—that is the problem.

KRAEPELIN: Yes, Your Honor.

BLEULER (*rising*): In my opinion, Professor Kraepelin—

JUDGE (*banging the gavel*): Professor Bleuler! Please, sir, this is not a debating society. You are an expert witness. Your testimony was accepted. You were thanked. You'll be paid. You cannot question other experts. Please, sir, be seated. (*Still angry, Bleuler sits down.*) You may sit down, Professor Kraepelin, thank you.

BINSWANGER (*coming to center stage*): Gentlemen, you have all read my ninety-four-page existential analysis of Ellen West. Therefore, let me be brief. I will summarize the world design of my patient. In Mrs. West's world, the complexity of an authentic experience has been reduced to the simplicity of the empty hole with the accompanying experience of emptiness. To fill up this void Mrs. West gorges and punishes herself in alternation. The consequence of this behavior is an increased awareness of lack of authenticity. It is this struggle between an authentic and an ersatz form of Being that has led Mrs. West to her recent experimenting with death. I would like to caution Ellen West, and share with my colleagues, my feeling that death itself can be a pseudo-experience, if it is only an escape from greed.

JUDGE: Did I understand correctly, Professor, that Mrs. West has a problem neither with thought nor with feeling but with authenticity?

BINSWANGER: Yes, Your Honor.

JUDGE: And she could die an unauthentic death?

BINSWANGER: She could.

JUDGE: And would that make it a different death?

BINSWANGER: From the existential point of view, certainly.

JUDGE (*puzzled*): Thank you, Professor. This has been most, but *most,* instructive. (*Indicates that he can sit down.*) And for the record, Professor, your qualifications?

BINSWANGER: I am Director of the Kreuzlingen Sanatorium.

(*During the previous period of darkness, Ellen's and Karl's chairs have been transformed into a courtroom dock. They hold hands, as if handcuffed to each other.*)

KARL (*Stands, Ellen's hand is pulled up with his*): What is the meaning of all this? Are you condemning or absolving her?

PSYCHIATRISTS (*in chorus*): M-hm . . .

KARL: What about me? Have all accusations against me been withdrawn?

PSYCHIATRISTS: M-hm . . .

KARL: Have I been absolved? Am I no longer responsible?

PSYCHIATRISTS: M-hm . . .

KARL: Is my slate clean? She did it all by herself?

PSYCHIATRISTS: M-hm . . .

KARL: Your Honor, I cannot accept freedom. I am guilty.

JUDGE: I am sorry, but I cannot interfere with their judgment. They own the legal right to fix labels. We have an agreement not to compete.

KARL: But I am responsible. Can *you,* at least, accept my guilt?

JUDGE: I am truly sorry, but as the lawyer for the defense your confession cannot be accepted. Plea denied.

KARL: Can I accuse the learned doctors?

JUDGE: Of what?

KARL: Of being her accomplices?

JUDGE: But how? They have only practiced their profession.

KARL: But each one of them gave a different diagnosis!

JUDGE: I know. I'm puzzled too.

KARL: And what will happen to Ellen?

(*The psychiatrists form a huddle at the table, consulting with each other. Ellen stands next to Karl and together they wait for a judgment.*)

BINSWANGER: Professor Bleuler and I are in agreement. First, we know very little about the treatment of schizophrenia. Second, we don't see the therapeutic use of Ellen West's remaining in the hospital. Third, if she leaves the hospital, she will commit suicide. Therefore a decision must be taken by her husband, Karl West.

KARL: The alternatives are life imprisonment or death?

PSYCHIATRISTS: M-hm . . .

KARL: And I am condemned to be the executioner?

PSYCHIATRISTS: M-hm . . .

(*Karl sits.*)

ELLEN (*still standing*): It's so beautiful. So clear! They have explained everything. Everything is explained! Why didn't I want to listen before? Now I know who I am, who I have become, what my world view is, in what world I am, how I fit in the world. It gives measurement to my dread, goals to my obsessions, faces to my demons. The world outside me is absolved and remains clean. I am right. I was always wrong. I don't have to fight any more. Everything has been labeled. I can decide now. My decision will be *mine*.

(*The judge rises slowly, removes his robe, folds it carefully, and places it on the chair. His wig follows.*)

JUDGE: Very confusing. Too many murderers. (*He returns to his seat in the audience.*)

(*The psychiatrists leave one by one. Ellen looks down at Karl, ruffles his hair in a loving gesture, then moves away, walking backward, still looking at him. Karl remains alone, looking into the audience with a vague, unfocused stare.*)

(*Lights to black*)

Scene 8

(*The room is just as it was, except that Karl wears a black mourning armband. He sits in the dock, holding a letter in his hand. He will not move during the scene. Voices envelop him—the voices have resonance and intensity, becoming a presence on the stage.*)

ELLEN'S VOICE (*light and vivacious*): You know, today I read a wonderful poem by Rilke. I think he captured the essence of our discussion.

Narcissus pined. The nearness of his being
kept on evaporating from his beauty
like scent of essenced heliotrope. But, seeing
that just to see himself was all his duty,

he loved back what had been in him before,
reconquered what the open wind had captured,
short-circuited perception, and, enraptured,
cancelled himself, and could exist no more.

KARL'S VOICE: You didn't understand. And they, with their learned voices, *certainly* didn't understand. You couldn't cancel yourself inside me. You exist in all the places we visited together. Whenever I encounter autumn leaves I'll feel my emptiness. In every apple I'll see the print of your teeth. Hiking on weekends I'll hear the echoes of your steps. In every bottle I'll see your brand of laxative. The chair in front of me is crying, unused. My arms feel estranged without your needy shape. You killed half of me. Why did you do it? Why did you condemn me to only half my sensations? The mark of Cain is branded on my forehead—it will be there forever.

(Far offstage, the voice of a cantor chants the Hebrew prayer for the dead. Karl weeps silently as the curtain falls.)

READER: Why did you write this play?

ELLEN WEST: I demanded a second hearing. I'm not pleased with the verdict on my life.

READER: What are *you* doing here? This space is reserved for the Author and me.

LORETTA GENOTTI: Let her talk. Her parents and her doctors stole her voice. She has the right to speak.

CARLO GENOTTI: Loretta, let her speak for herself. She's not your sister.

LORETTA: Of course she is.

MARGHERITA GENOTTI: That's impossible. She's not even Italian!

READER: Will you please control these people? I asked you a question.

AUTHOR: I agree with Ellen.

MILTON WEST: You can't mean that!

MARTHA WEST: I thought you were on our side! You have a daughter!

KARL: He thinks the Wests are a circle, with no sides.

READER: If you agree with Ellen, isn't that taking a linear position?

PIERRE RIVIÈRE: I think he means that he agrees with the need of silenced voices to be heard.

READER: Is that a correct interpretation of your play?

MRS. OBUTU: You talk like an English magistrate. Precisely how much pain must you endure before you have the right to cry?

AUTHOR: I never thought about it until Ellen said it but, yes, I feel like the judge of an appellate court. Perhaps I should have called the book "A Second Hearing."

TOM: If ours was a second hearing, it was still in a capitalist courtroom, where justice is only a label for . . .

JANE: He did amplify the woman's voice.

TOM: That was a trick to destroy the commune.

READER: May I ask a question?

ELLEN WEST: No. This is my only chance, but this time I'm going to have the last word.

AUTHOR: But . . .

ELLEN: Not this time. No.

Works Cited

Bass, Ellen, and Louise Thornton, eds., *I Never Told Anyone: Writings by Women Survivors of Child Sexual Abuse* (New York: Harper and Row, 1983), pp. 42, 14.

Binswanger, Ludwig, "The Case of Ellen West: An Anthropological-Clinical Study," in Rollo May, Ernest Angel, and Henri F. Ellenberger, eds., *Existence: A New Dimension in Psychiatry and Psychology* (New York: Basic Books, 1958), pp. 237–364.

Cooper, David, *The Death of the Family* (New York: Pantheon, 1970).

Foucault, Michel, ed., *I, Pierre Rivière, having slaughtered my mother, my sister, and my brother . . . A Case of Parricide in the 19th Century,* translated by Frank Jellinek (New York: Pantheon Books, a Division of Random House, Inc., copyright 1975). Quotations from pp. 54–55, 209, 55, 56, 57, 61, 66, 74, 106, 112, 124, 108, 105.

Francke, Linda Bird, *Growing Up Divorced* (New York: Linden Press/Simon and Schuster, 1983), p. 117.

Friedenberg, Edgar Z., *R. D. Laing* (New York: Viking Press, 1973), p. 70.

Goldstein, Joseph, et al., *Before the Best Interests of the Child* (Glencoe: Free Press, 1980), pp. 143–144.

Gruber, Alan R., *Foster Home Care in Massachusetts* (Boston: Commonwealth of Massachusetts, Governor's Commission on Adoption and Foster Care, 1973).

Health, Education, and Welfare, U.S. Department of, *Child Abuse and Neglect: An Overview of the Problems,* vol. 1 (Washington, D.C., 1975), p. 50.

Marx, Emanuel, *The Social Context of Violent Behavior* (London: Routledge and Kegan Paul, 1976).

Minuchin, Salvador, "The Use of an Ecological Framework in the Treatment of a Child," in E. James Anthony and Cyrille Koupernik, eds., *The Child in His Family* (New York: Wiley, 1970), pp. 41–57.

———— Braulio Montalvo, et al., *Families of the Slums: An Exploration of Their Structure and Treatment* (New York: Basic Books, 1967).

———— Bernice Rosman and Lester Baker, *Psychosomatic Families: Anorexia Nervosa in Context* (Cambridge: Harvard University Press, 1978).

Stone, Lawrence, *The Family, Sex and Marriage: England, 1500–1800* (New York: Harper and Row, 1977).

Wallerstein, Judith S., and Joan B. Kelly, *Surviving the Breakup: How Children and Parents Cope with Divorce* (New York: Basic Books, 1980).